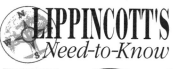

ECG

FACTS

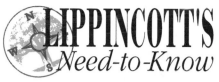

LIPPINCOTT'S
Need-to-Know
ECG
FACTS

Mary Jo Boyer, RN, DNSc.

PROFESSOR AND ASSOCIATE DEAN

Allied Health and Nursing
Delaware County Community College
Media, Pennsylvania

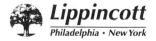

Lippincott
Philadelphia · New York

Acquisitions Editor: Lisa Stead
Sponsoring Editor: Gail Feinberg
Project Editor: Erika Kors
Production Manager: Helen Ewan
Production Coordinator: Nannette Winski
Design Coordinator: Lisa Caro

9 8 7 6 5 4 3 2 1

Library of Congress Cataloging-in-Publications Data

Boyer, Mary Jo.
    Lippincott's need-to-know ECG facts / Mary Jo Boyer.
        p. cm.—(Lippincott's need-to-know)
    ISBN 0-397-55461-3 (alk. paper)
    1. Electrocardiography.   2. Cardiovascular system—Diseases—Nursing.   I. Title.   II. Series.
    [DNLM: 1. Arrhythmia—diagnosis.   2. Arrythmia—physiopathology.   3. Electrocardiography.   WG 330 B791L 1997
RC683.5.E5B66 1997]
616.1'207547—dc21   97-9089
for Library of Congress   CIP

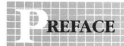

PREFACE

This reference book contains all the information you will "need-to-know" to perform an electrocardiogram accurately, to identify commonly occurring arrhythmias and determine arrhythmia origin, to recognize deflections caused by artifacts, and to distinguish between an occasional normal arrhythmia and a potentially life-threatening one.

This book is divided into six units. The first unit (Chapters 1–3) serves as a review of the heart's anatomy and physiology, its electrical conduction and the basic components of an electrocardiogram. Chapter 1 presents the heart's electrical conduction system with an entire section devoted to the cardiac cell. Chapter 2 focuses on the electrocardiogram (ECG) and the rationale for electrode (lead) placement. Standard, augmented, and precordial leads are discussed and placement positions illustrated. In Chapter 3 the basic components (lines and deflections) of the electrocardiogram (waveforms, intervals, segments, and complexes) are explained relative to their shape, appearance, and frequency of occurrence. Rhythm strips are provided to practice identification of the ECG components. An answer key that begins at the end of Chapter 14 provides detailed analysis of each rhythm strip.

Unit II (Chapters 4 and 5) covers the fundamental techniques of estimating rhythm regularity and calculating heart rate. The concepts of time/rate and amplitude/voltage are presented. The unit ends with a detailed, step-by-step explanation of how to perform an electrocardiogram. Adult and pediatric applications are also presented. Chapter 4 ends with the first of a series of

"Practice Analysis of Rhythm Strips" exercises that are provided to reinforce content just learned.

Unit III begins the in-depth coverage of arrhythmia recognition and interpretation. Chapters 6 through 8 cover the most common sinus and atrial arrhythmias and atrioventricular junctional arrhythmias and blocks. Each arrhythmia is explained and outlined according to etiology, symptomatology, primary treatment goals, and unique ECG pattern characteristics (rate, rhythm, conduction, P waves, PR interval, and QRS complex). A sample rhythm strip is provided for each arrhythmia presented in detail.

Unit IV covers arrhythmias and cardiac disease affecting the ventricles, the most serious of all arrhythmias. The significance of six ventricular arrhythmias is presented in Chapter 9. A distinction between ischemia and myocardial tissue injury is made in Chapter 10, where angina pectoris is compared to myocardial infarction. Illustrations are provided for the four anatomical sites for myocardial infarction and ECG interpretation specific to lead placement is reviewed.

Unit V covers miscellaneous arrhythmias. Chapter 11 presents arrhythmias caused by conduction abnormalities associated with four types of bundle branch blocks. Arrhythmias caused by electrolyte disturbances, primarily potassium and calcium, and three popular antiarrhythmic drugs (digitalis, procainamide, and quinidine) is presented in Chapter 12.

Unit VI covers pacemaker therapy and continuous cardiac monitoring. Chapter 13 presents the purpose and function of internal and external pacemakers and the difference between temporary and permanent pacemakers. Rhythm interpretation is explained relative to ECG patterns specific to pacemaker activity. Chapter 14 reviews the purpose of continuous cardiac monitoring and electrode placement for telemetry monitoring. The ncept of artifacts is reviewed and four rhythm strips provide sample ECG patterns influenced by different types of artifacts.

It is the author's intent that this book be user-friendly, easy to read, and easy to comprehend. Toward that goal, the language has been simplified and the script written in the personal tense. This book is intended to present "need-to-know" information about ECG's for any level of health care provider, from a patient care technician to a registered nurse. It is the author's intent that this essential information will make the task of performing and analyzing ECGs easier, thus improving the quality of patient care delivery.

ACKNOWLEDGMENTS

Special thanks are extended to Lisa Stead, Editor, for her vision and leadership during the development of this textbook. Recognition is also given to Gary Gustin, RN, BS, instructor at Delaware County Community College and occupational nurse, a respected clinical practitioner who teaches allied health and nursing students how to perform and interpret ECGs. Gary reviewed this textbook from the perspective of an educator, providing constructive criticism about reading level and applicability for students as well as those currently working in the field. Appreciation is also extended to Leslie Mickles, RN, MSN, CCRN, clinical educator-professional services at Crozer-Chester Medical Center in Chester, Pennsylvania. Leslie reviewed this textbook for the accuracy and comprehensiveness of content considered essential for current clinical practice in a variety of settings (ie., acute care, long-term care, and/or home care). Kathy Campitelli should also be recognized for her assistance with typing, especially with the development of charts used throughout. As with any book, the final manuscript is a team effort and everyone's contributions are sincerely appreciated and recognized.

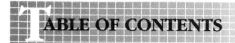

TABLE OF CONTENTS

Unit I

The Heart, Its Electrophysiology and Electrocardiographic Patterns

Unit II

Fundamental Techniques of Determining Heart Rate and Rhythm and Performing an ECG

Unit III

Arrhythmias of Sinus and Atrial Origin

Unit IV
Arrhythmias and Cardiac Disease
Affecting the Ventricles

Unit V
Miscellaneous Arrhythmias

Unit VI
Pacemaker Therapy and Continuous
Cardiac Monitoring

LIST OF CHARTS

CHAPTER 4

CHAPTER 10

CHAPTER 13

LIST OF ABBREVIATIONS

AV	atrioventricular
CAD	coronary artery disease
CHF	congestive heart failure
CNS	central nervous system
CPR	cardiopulmonary resuscitation
ECG	electrocardiogram, graph, graphic
IV	intravenous
MI	myocardial infarction
OTC	over-the-counter
SA	sinoatrial

LIPPINCOTT'S
Need-to-Know
ECG
FACTS

Unit 1

The Heart, Its Electrophysiology and Electrocardiographic Patterns

This unit reviews the heart's general structure, physiologic function, and electrical conduction system. The electrophysiology of the cardiac cell and its inherent ability to depolarize and conduct electrical impulses are presented as foundation concepts. The structure and significance of the coronary arteries are reviewed specific to conduction interruptions secondary to tissue ischemia and injury.

The use of the ECG as an assessment tool is described in detail. The concept of a vector, the direction and magnitude of the heart's electrical current flow, is correlated to ECG patterns. The rationale for electrode and lead placements is explained.

This unit ends with a comprehensive presentation on the components of the ECG. Waveforms, intervals, segments, and the QRS complex are explained in detail relative to the deflections and lines produced on ECG graph paper.

This unit provides the foundation knowledge necessary to move to the next step—learning how to perform an ECG, estimate rhythm and calculate heart rate. Take as much time as you need to learn, review, and understand these basic concepts. This information establishes the framework necessary for you to understand how to analyze and interpret ECGs.

CHAPTER ONE
THE HEART AND ITS ELECTRICAL CONDUCTION

The Heart

The heart, which is a muscular organ positioned between the second and sixth ribs, lies behind the sternum. The bottom tip of the heart points to the left and is called the *apex*. The heart's major function is to pump blood throughout the cardiovascular system. It is stimulated to contract and relax, in an organized rhythm, by electricity and chemical agents.

The heart's surface is divided into four areas: anterior (front), posterior (back), inferior (bottom), and lateral (side) (Fig. 1-1). It is important to memorize these positions because these terms will be used throughout the book, especially when identifying specific areas of myocardial tissue damage.

The heart has four compartments or chambers. The two upper and smaller chambers, the right and left atria, are divided by a wall, the interatrial septum. The two lower chambers, the right and left ventricles, are divided by a thicker wall, the interventricular septum.

The right atrium receives deoxygenated blood from the body after oxygen has been extracted and used by the body. The right atrium contracts and pumps venous blood into the right ventricle, which, in turn, contracts and pumps the blood into the lungs where it receives oxygen. Blood, rich in nutrients and oxygen (oxygenated), then enters the left atrium from the lungs, is pumped into the

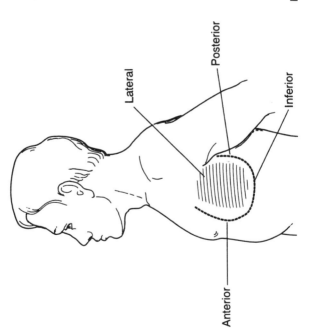

Figure 1-1. The heart's surfaces.

right ventricle, and is then pumped out of the right ventricle into the aorta and the body (arterial blood) (Fig. 1-2). The cardiac muscle forming the walls of these chambers is called the myocardium.

The four heart valves have the primary function of regulating blood flow, in one direction, throughout the heart and lungs. The *tricuspid valve* separates the right atrium and the right ventricle and the *pulmonic valve* separates the right ventricle and the pulmonary artery. The *mitral valve* separates the left atrium and the left ventricle and the *aortic valve* separates the left ventricle and the aorta. It is important to understand the function of each valve when working with the heart; however, for purposes of this book, little reference will be made to these valves.

The *coronary arteries* supply the heart with blood. Both the right and left coronary arteries arise from the aorta. The right coronary artery supplies blood to the right atrium and right ventricle, the SA and AV nodes, and the inferior and posterior walls of the left ventricle. The left coronary artery separates into the anterior descending branch and the circumflex branch. The anterior wall of the left ventricle is supplied by the anterior descending branch and the lateral side of the ventricle is supplied by the circumflex branch. When blood flow is restricted or diminished, ischemia (decreased tissue oxygenation), or necrosis (cellular tissue death) occurs. These tissue changes are discussed in more detail in Chapter 10 where the medical conditions of angina pectoris and MI are presented.

Cardiac Cells

The heart, made up of cardiac cells, is stimulated by electrical conduction to mechanically contract and relax, in an organized rhythm. The *automaticity* of these cells refers to their ability to generate

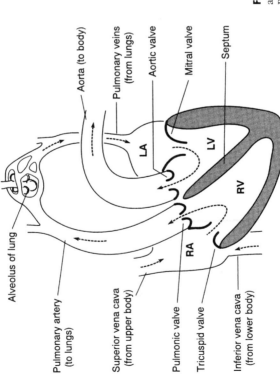

Figure 1-2. The heart's structure. LA, left atrium; LV, left ventricle; RA, right atrium; RV, right ventricle.

and transmit an electrical impulse. Cardiac cells are divided into three types of specialized cells. *Pacemaker* cells, the electrical power source of the heart, generate the electrical impulses. Pacemaker cells are located in the upper wall of the right atrium in the SA node. These cells fire at a rate of 60 to 100 times per minute and help set the basic pace for the rest of the heart. *Conducting* cells transmit impulses throughout the myocardium from the atrial nodes to the ventricles. *Myocardial* cells deliver blood to the body by contracting and relaxing. Every cardiac cell is surrounded by and filled with a fluid that contains positively and negatively charged ions (ie, calcium, potassium, sodium), which carry the electrical impulses that stimulate the heart to beat. Cardiac cells, while resting, have negatively charged ions on the inside and positively charged ions on the outside (Fig. 1-3). At rest, sodium and calcium exist in larger amounts outside the cell with potassium in larger amounts inside the cell.

The cardiac cell's receptivity to an electrical stimulus is known as the cell's *excitability*. When an electrical current stimulates a cardiac cell, positive ions on the outside move rapidly inside the cell

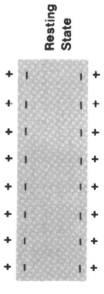

Resting State

Figure 1-3. Resting state of a cardiac cell prior to depolarization.

7

at the same time that negative ions on the inside move rapidly to the outside (Fig. 1-4). Sodium and calcium start to move into the cell while potassium moves outside. This is the beginning of *depolarization*.

This wave of depolarization continues rhythmically from one end of the cell to the other, until complete depolarization occurs, with potassium primarily outside the cell and sodium and calcium inside the cell. This impulse transfer occurs because cardiac cells have the property of *conductivity*.

Depolarization and Repolarization

Depolarization is the basic, fundamental electrical activity of the heart. This progressive movement of electricity, from one cardiac cell to another, occurs until the entire heart is affected. This movement occurs so rapidly that it appears to happen all at one time. A second wave of depolarization occurs only after the first wave of depolarization is complete. This period of time is known as the *absolute refractory period*.

This wave or movement of an electrical current can be detected by electrodes placed on the body and transmitted to an ECG machine.

The absolute refractory period is that phase of the cardiac cycle where the ventricular myocardium will not respond to any stimulus, no matter how strong. On a normal ECG recording, this period extends from the beginning of the QRS complex (ventricular depolarization) to the beginning of the T wave (early ventricular repolarization).

After depolarization is complete, the cell begins to repolarize, or return to its resting state. This transition is initiated at the end of the cell that was just depolarized. During repolarization, positive

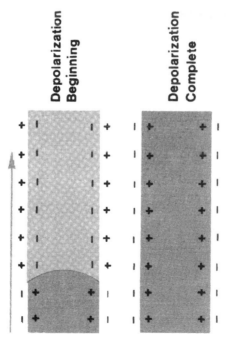

Figure 1-4. Depolarization of a cardiac cell.

ions move back to the outside of the cell as the negative ions return to the inside (Fig. 1-5). Repolarization is complete when the cell is in a resting state waiting for the next wave of depolarization.

During repolarization, a *relative refractory period* occurs. This is the phase of the cardiac cycle where early ventricular repolarization begins (beginning of the T wave) and proceeds through late ventricular depolarization. This is a dangerous part of the cardiac cycle because some cardiac cells are

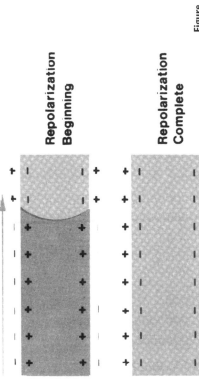

Figure 1-5. Repolarization of a cardiac cell.

depolarizing while others are repolarizing. A strong internal or external stimulus occurring at this time can cause an abnormal ventricular conduction that can lead to a fatal arrhythmia.

During repolarization, beginning near the end of the T wave, and ending at the beginning of the QRS complex, the cardiac cycle goes through a *diminished refractory period*. During this time, the myocardium is sensitive to any strong stimulus that can produce a premature depolarization. If this happens, the contraction will result in diminished cardiac output because repolarization is not long enough to permit adequate chamber refilling.

The Electrical Conduction System

You have now reviewed how the heart pumps blood throughout the body when cardiac cells contract as a result of electrical stimulation. You have also learned how each cardiac cell depolarizes and repolarizes, transferring energy throughout cardiac cells. The cardiac cells are part of a larger electrical conduction system that has five subcomponents (Fig. 1-6). The rest of this chapter details how electrical impulse transmission results in myocardial contractions.

The SA Node

The SA node, also known as the *pacemaker of the heart*, is located in the upper right atrial wall just below the opening of the superior vena cava. The SA node, oval in shape, fires electrical impulses at a rate of 60 to 100 beats/min through internodal pathways, causing both atria to contract. The

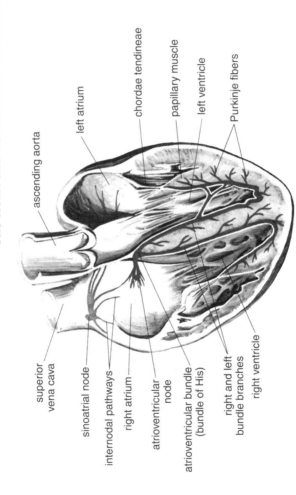

Figure 1-6. The heart's electrical conduction system.

SA node sets the pace for the heart's electrical conduction system and can initiate impulses independently.

The AV Node

The AV node is located on the right side of the interatrial septum near the tricuspid valve. The AV node receives the cardiac impulse from the SA node, and after a slight pause, relays the impulse to the AV bundle, the Bundle of His. This delayed transmission of the impulse at the AV node provides time for the atria to contract so blood can completely fill the ventricles.

The Bundle of His

The bundle of His is a cluster of specialized muscle fibers located in the superior portion of the interventricular septum. The impulse travels rapidly through the His bundle to the bundle branches.

The Bundle Branches

The His bundle is divided into the right and left bundle branches located along the right and left side of the interventricular septum. The cardiac impulse travels down both branches and passes into the conduction myofibers (Purkinje fibers)

The Purkinje Fibers

Each network of right and left bundle branches spreads out into a network of tiny myofibers within the ventricular myocardium. The cardiac impulse is rapidly delivered to the apex of the ventricular myocardium and then around and upward through the rest of the myocardium, stimulating ventricular myocardial contraction.

This concludes the fundamental information you need to know about the heart and its electrical conduction properties. You should now understand how electrical activity can be transmitted to the surface of the body and picked up by electrodes. These electrodes are connected to wires that transmit electricity to the ECG machine so patterns can be recorded on ECG paper. Each line, waveform, segment, interval, and complex is reflected on strips of ECG paper.

CHAPTER TWO
THE ECG

The ECG

The heart produces electrical activity with every heartbeat. This electrical activity can be detected on the skin's surface and recorded by using a special machine known as an electrocardiograph. The recording of the heart's electrical activity, on a strip of graph paper, is an ECG. This recording is possible through the use of standard bipolar electrodes that transmit and amplify the heart's electrical activity, through conductive wires, to the machine, which produces 12 different angles of looking at the heart. These electrodes are commonly referred to as "leads."

Vectors

A vector refers to the direction and magnitude of the heart's electrical current flow that creates the waveform deflection on the ECG. A vector is specifically what the ECG electrodes record and translate into wave patterns that are seen on the ECG. A vector points out the *direction* of atrial or ventricular depolarization waves in the heart.

Arrows can be used to illustrate vector and mean vector direction. When these vector arrows are superimposed on a drawing of the heart, it is easy to see how the wave of depolarization proceeds from the atria to the ventricles. It is also obvious that these electrical forces move progressively from the right to the left, from atrial depolarization to ventricular depolarization.

The term *mean vector* is used to identify the average of depolarization waves in one section of the heart. The *mean P vector* represents the average direction and magnitude of both right and left atrial depolarization (Fig. 2-1). The *mean QRS vector* represents the average direction and magnitude of both right and left ventricular depolarization (Fig. 2-2). The average direction of a mean vector is called the *mean axis*. It is identified *only in the frontal plane*.

ECG Electrodes (Leads)

The heart's electrical conduction system initiates the cardiac impulse in the SA node. This impulse stimulates the waves of atrial and ventricular depolarization and repolarization that can be recorded and translated into the wave patterns seen on the ECG. The direction and magnitude of these wave patterns depend on proper ECG electrode (lead) placement.

The ECG electrodes are placed on designated areas of the body so different pictures of the heart's electrical activity can be translated into wave patterns and recorded on ECG graph paper. Before you learn where and how to place each electrode, you should understand why the leads must be placed in standard, anatomic positions.

(text continues on page 19)

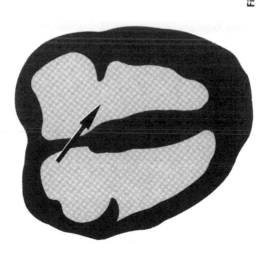

Figure 2-1. The mean P vector.

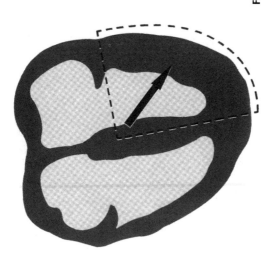

Figure 2-2. The mean QRS vector.

The ECG is recorded by using either a single channel or a 12-lead ECG machine. With the 12-lead ECG, there are six leads for the arms and legs (limb leads); three are standard, three are augmented. The electrode on the right leg *acts as a ground* for all leads. The three standard leads are *bipolar* because each has a negative and a positive electrode. The augmented leads are *unipolar* because they are composed of only one positive electrode. Because of the arrangement of these unipolar leads, voltage is low and must be *augmented* by the ECG machine to increase the electrical potential.

The 12-lead ECG allows for viewing specific regions of the heart, each at a unique angle, so arrhythmias can be identified, cardiac function analyzed, and pathology diagnosed. The angles are viewed from two different surfaces—a *vertical* or *frontal* view and a *horizontal* or *transverse* view. These views are called "planes," points of reference by which an angle of the heart can be examined.

The *six limb leads* allow you to view the heart from the *frontal view* or *plane*. These leads analyze the electrical impulses of depolarization and repolarization that move up and down and left to right across the chest. The *six precordial leads* view the heart from the *horizontal plane*. These leads analyze the electrical impulses of depolarization and repolarization from the viewpoint of looking down at the heart from the top of the body.

Each lead determines a different view of the heart because each lead looks at the heart from a different angle. Each lead records the *average* current flow at a specific time. The diagram in Figure 2-3 illustrates how angles are formed by specific lead placements. Consider the frontal view of the body. Draw a straight line across the body from right to left. Then draw a line, from top to bottom, to intersect this line at midpoint. Label these lines with degrees of measurement enclosed within a 360° circle with the heart at the intersection of both lines.

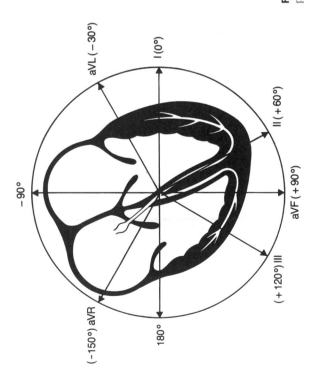

Figure 2-3. Angles of orientation for lead placement.

Standard Leads

The three standard leads are bipolar, each having one positive and one negative electrode. The difference in the electrical potential between these electrodes is what is recorded on the ECG. These leads are also referred to as limb leads.

When referring to these three leads:

Lead I: Right arm is negative and left arm is positive.
Lead II: Right arm is negative and left leg is positive.
Lead III: Left arm is negative and left leg is positive.

LIMB LEAD I

This lead measures the electrical conductivity between the right arm (designated negative) and the left arm (designated positive). Because this lead lies on a straight line, running from right to left, there is no angle of orientation when assessing this recording on the ECG graph paper (Fig. 2–4**A**).

LIMB LEAD II

This lead measures the electrical conductivity between the right arm (designated negative) and the left leg (designated positive). This lead runs downward from negative to positive, creating a 60° angle of visualization (Fig. 2–4**B**)

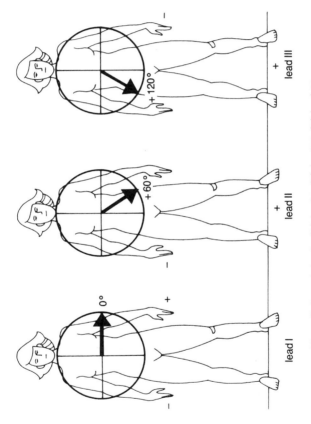

Figure 2-4. Limb leads. **(A)** lead I; **(B)** lead II; **(C)** lead III.

LIMB LEAD III

This lead measures the electrical conductivity between the left arm (designated negative) and the left leg (designated positive). The line runs downward from negative to positive, creating a 120° angle of visualization (Fig. 2-4C).

Augmented Leads

These three leads are unipolar. Each lead has one positive electrode, which can be for the left arm, left leg, or right arm. Because of lead arrangement, voltage is low and needs to be augmented by the ECG machine. When referring to augmented leads, each letter refers to a specific term.

REMEMBER

a means *augmented.*
V means *voltage.*
R means *right arm.*
L means *left arm.*
F means *foot or legs, usually the left.*

LEAD aVL

This lead is designed by making the *left arm* positive while all other limbs are negative. Therefore, electrical activity or augmented voltage is recorded toward the direction of the left arm, creating a −30° angle (Fig. 2-5A).

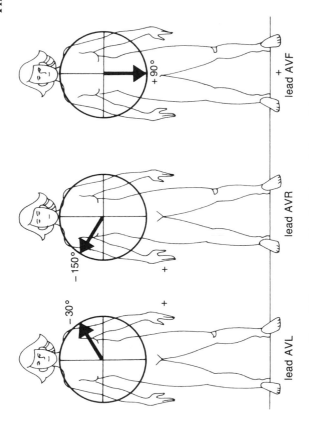

Figure 2-5. Augmented leads. **(A)** aVL; **(B)** aVR; **(C)** aVF.

LEAD aVR

This lead is designed by making the *right arm* positive while all other limbs are negative. Therefore, electrical activity or augmented voltage is recorded toward the direction of the right arm, creating a −150° angle (Fig. 2-5**B**)

LEAD aVF

This lead is designed by making the *legs or left foot* positive while all other limbs are negative. Therefore, electrical activity or augmented voltage is recorded toward the direction of the left leg or bottom of the heart, creating a +90° angle (Fig. 2-5**C**).

Precordial Leads

The six precordial leads, also referred to as chest leads or "V" leads, are all positive electrodes. An electrical potential difference is created by the body. These leads form angles of orientation using the same intersection of lines within a 360° circle. The angles of orientation created are angles viewed by looking down on the heart.

REMEMBER

✓ V_1 and V_2 leads lie over the *right ventricle*.
V_3 and V_4 leads lie over the *interventricular septum*.
V_5 and V_6 leads lie over the *left ventricle*.

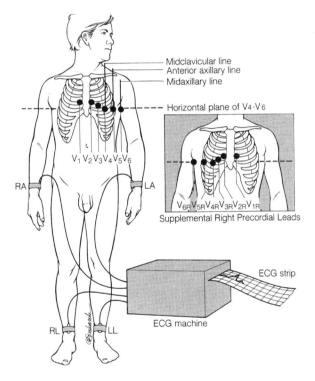

Figure 2-6. Precordial lead placement.

Precordial lead V$_1$ is placed to the right of the sternum at the fourth intercostal space (between the ribs). The angle created is +120°. Precordial lead V$_2$ is placed to the left of the sternum, immediately opposite V$_1$, at the fourth intercostal space. The angle created is +90°. Precordial lead V$_3$ is placed midway between V$_2$ and V$_4$. The angle created is +75°. Precordial lead V$_4$ is placed at the fifth intercostal space, left midclavicular line. The angle created is +60°. Precordial lead V$_5$ is placed between V$_4$ and V$_6$, at the fifth intercostal space, at the left anterior axillary line. The angle created is +30°. Precordial lead V$_6$ is placed at the fifth intercostal space on the left midaxillary line, just below the armpit. The placement of V$_4$, V$_5$, and V$_6$ are directly along the same horizontal plane. There is no angle created (Fig. 2-6).

Correct anatomic placement of leads is essential to obtain an accurate "picture" or ECG recording of the heart's activity. This picture will be interpreted and the information used to diagnose and manage cardiac disorders. Chapter 3 focuses on the meaning of waveforms, intervals, segments, and complexes relative to identifying various ECG patterns.

CHAPTER THREE

ECG COMPONENTS: WAVEFORMS, INTERVALS, SEGMENTS, AND COMPLEXES

A normal cycle of cardiac electrical activity encompasses atrial and ventricular contraction (systole) and relaxation (diastole). Each cycle of systole and diastole produces the lines and waves seen on the standard ECG. The ECG pattern produced depends on the arrangement of positive and negative electrodes. In this chapter, you will learn the meaning of the basic components of the ECG pattern as seen on an ECG tracing. You may need to refer back to Chapter 2 to review lead placement as each component is explained.

The Baseline or Isoelectric Line

The baseline or isoelectric line is a straight line on the ECG paper where the positive and negative electrical charges are balanced so there is no deflection. This isoelectric line occurs between the waveforms of the ECG pattern, usually between the T wave and the P wave (Fig. 3-1).

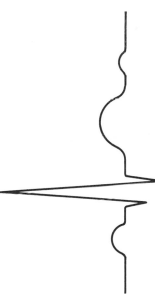

Figure 3-1. The baseline or isoelectric line.

Waveforms

Waveforms are representations of the electrical activity generated by the depolarization and repolarization of the atria and ventricles. If electrical current flow is *moving toward* a lead, then a *positive* deflection will be seen on the ECG. current flowing *away from* a lead will cause a *negative* deflection. Waveforms that are positive create upward deflections above the isoelectric line; negative waveforms create downward deflections below the isoelectric line. Waveforms that are both above and below the line are called *biphasic*. Waveforms can be curved or pointed. Figure 3-2 compares waveforms and the

29

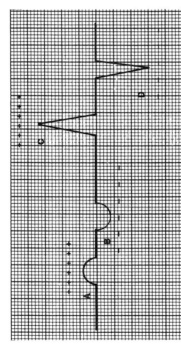

Figure 3-2. Waveforms, lines, and electrical activity.

isoelectric line. The letters (A, B, C, and D) reflect the movement of positive and negative ions as the waves of depolarization and repolarization move throughout the heart.

The P Wave

Electrical impulses originating in the SA node trigger atrial depolarization. The shape and deflection of the P wave gives information about the origin of the impulse and any atrial pathology. The normal P wave is no more than 0.1 second in duration and 2.5 mm high (Fig. 3-3).

ATRIAL DEPOLARIZATION

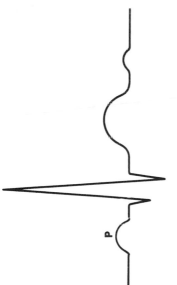

Figure 3-3. The P Wave, normally upright and slightly rounded.

The direction of electrical current flow, from the SA node to the AV node, is from the right side of the chest toward the left arm. Therefore, current direction is from negative to positive. The P wave, the first deflection in the normal ECG pattern, represents the time it takes for the electrical impulse to successfully complete atrial depolarization. The P wave, which is normally small and curved, will have a *positive deflection* and be its tallest when seen from the frontal view in lead II. Because the wave of atrial depolarization is moving at right angles in leads III and aVL, this deflection will be very small or nonexistent in these leads. Lead aVR records atrial depolarization from the completely opposite direction; the P wave will have a negative deflection on the ECG strip in this lead (Fig. 3-4). From the horizontal view, atrial depolarization is recorded as a positive deflection in precordial leads V_5 and V_6; it is biphasic in lead V_1.

The T Wave

Ventricular repolarization, which immediately follows ventricular depolarization, is represented by the T wave. The T wave is the first upward deflection after the QRS complex. Its shape is rounded and its duration is taller and wider than the P wave. T waves also exhibit the most variability, being sensitive to a variety of hormonal and physiologic factors. The T wave is usually 5 to 10 mm in height (Fig. 3-5).

The direction of electrical current flow is opposite the approaching wave of depolarization, which usually generates a positive deflection on the ECG. T waves are positive in the same leads that have positive QRS complexes (tall R waves) and negative in the same leads that have negative QRS complexes (inverted R waves). These leads are I, II, and V_3 to V_6. The V_2 lead is an exception to this. The T wave is shown in all leads in Figures 3-6 and 3-7.

The U Wave

After ventricular repolarization and before atrial depolarization, an isoelectric line can sometimes reflect a U wave (Fig. 3-8). The U wave is of the same deflection as the T wave but the height of its rounded shape is similar to the P wave. The U wave is thought to represent late repolarization of the Purkinje fibers in the ventricles. Figures 3-9 and 3-10 show an ECG strip with and without a U wave.

(text continues on page 39)

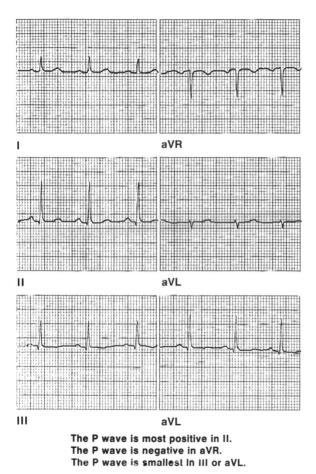

I   aVR

II   aVL

III   aVL

The P wave is most positive in II.
The P wave is negative in aVR.
The P wave is smallest in III or aVL.

Figure 3-4. Normal P wave configurations.

VENTRICULAR REPOLARIZATION

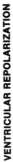
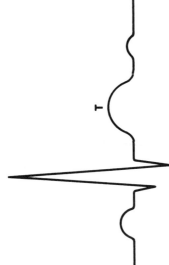

Figure 3-5. The T wave, normally upright and slightly rounded.

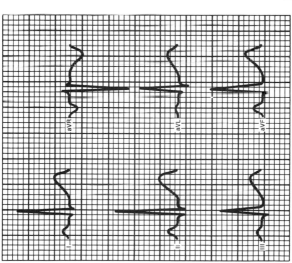

Figure 3-6. Normal T waves in standard and augmented leads.

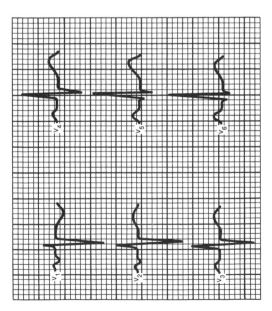

Figure 3-7. Normal T waves in the precordial leads.

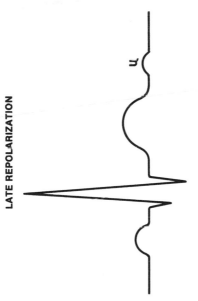

Figure 3-8. Normal U wave in same direction as P wave.

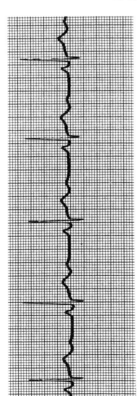

Figure 3-9. ECG with a U wave present.

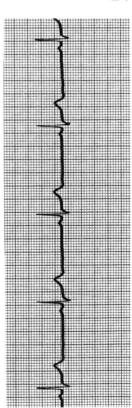

Figure 3-10. ECG without a U wave.

Intervals

The term *interval* refers to the length of a particular wave plus the isoelectric line that follows it; the length of an interval ends when another wave begins. An interval is named using the letters of both waves on either side. Intervals contain waves.

The PR Interval

The PR interval is the length of the baseline from the beginning of the P wave to the beginning of the QRS complex. This time interval represents atrial depolarization and the time it takes for the impulse to be delayed at the AV node before ventricular depolarization (Fig. 3-11). The PR interval is normally about 0.12 to 0.20 second in duration.

The QT Interval

The QT interval is the length of the baseline from the beginning of the QRS complex to the end of the T wave. This time interval represents ventricular depolarization and repolarization. In the presence of a U wave, the QT interval should be measured from the beginning of the QRS complex to the end of the U wave (see Fig. 3-11).

Segments

The term *segment* refers to the baseline between the end of one wave and the beginning of the next wave. It is always straight, not deflected upward or downward, and named by the wave that precedes or follows it. Segments are the lines between the waves.

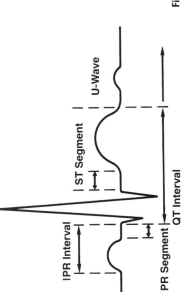

Figure 3-11. Intervals and segments.

The ST Segment

The ST segment is the length of the baseline between the end of the S wave of the QRS complex and the beginning of the T wave. This segment represents the time from the end of ventricular depolarization to the end of ventricular repolarization. It is electrically neutral (see Fig. 3-11).

The PR Segment

The PR segment is also an electrically neutral segment. It represents the delay in conduction from atrial depolarization to the beginning of ventricular depolarization (see Fig. 3-11).

The Complex

An ECG has only one *complex*, the QRS complex. A complex occurs when one wave follows another, without any intervals, segments, or isoelectric lines between them. The QRS complex is composed of three waves: the Q wave, the R wave, and the S wave.

The QRS Complex

The QRS complex represents ventricular depolarization. This complex is usually the most striking feature of the ECG because of its variability and because the R waveform can cover a significant distance. The normal QRS complex consists of three waveforms. The complex begins with its first downward deflection known as the Q wave. This is followed by an upward deflection called the R wave.

The next downward deflection after the R wave is called an S wave. With certain arrhythmias, an extra R wave, R prime (R'), and an extra S wave, S prime (S'), will occur. All ventricular complexes are referred to as a QRS complex, even if every wave is not present in all complexes (Fig. 3-12). The QRS complex is normally 0.04 to 0.10 second in duration.

Depolarization begins in the interventricular septum and proceeds in a left-to-right direction. Since this electrical movement is directed *away from* the positive electrodes of leads I, II, aVL, V$_5$, and V$_6$,

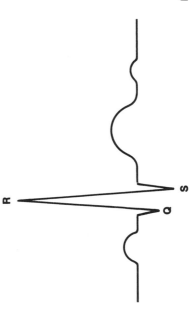

VENTRICULAR DEPOLARIZATION

Figure 3-12. The QRS complex.

an initial tiny negative deflection is seen as a Q wave in these leads. This wave is followed by completion of right ventricular depolarization when the current moves downward and toward the left.

A positive deflection or R wave is recorded along with a negative deflection (S wave) in leads I, II, aVL, and V_3 through V_6. Electrical activity moves toward the left as the left ventricle completely depolarizes. Tall, positive deflections (R waves) are seen in the left heart leads and negative deflections (S waves) are in the right heart leads. Figures 3-13 and 3-14 show examples of QRS complexes in all leads.

Unit Summary

In the previous chapters you reviewed the basic anatomy and physiology of the heart, the heart's electrical conduction system, and the meaning of the components of the ECG. Before advancing to the next step of identifying abnormal rhythms and specific arrhythmias, you need to understand the concepts of time and voltage, learn how to determine rate and rhythm, and be knowledgeable about the procedure for accurately taking an ECG. These topics are presented in Unit II.

Practice Analysis of Rhythm Strips

On each of the eight sample rhythm strips (pps. 46–48) identify and label each waveform (P, Q, R, S, T, and U). You may write directly on each strip. Use a pencil first. After checking your answer in the answer key and making any corrections, you can change the labeling to ink and use these rhythm strips later for reference or review.

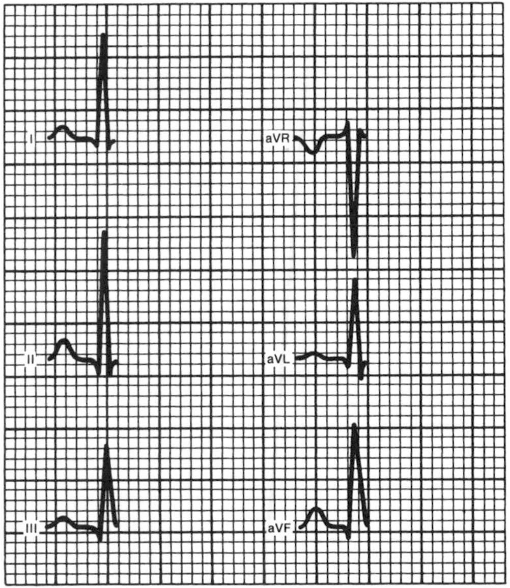

Figure 3-13. Normal QRS complexes in standard and augmented leads.

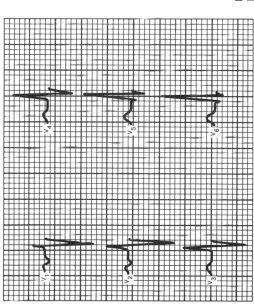

Figure 3-14. Normal QRS complexes in the precordial leads.

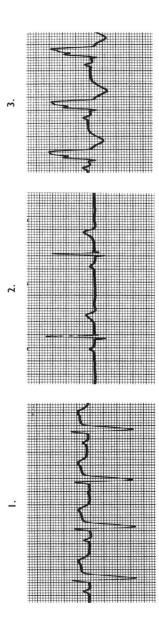

1.

2.

3.

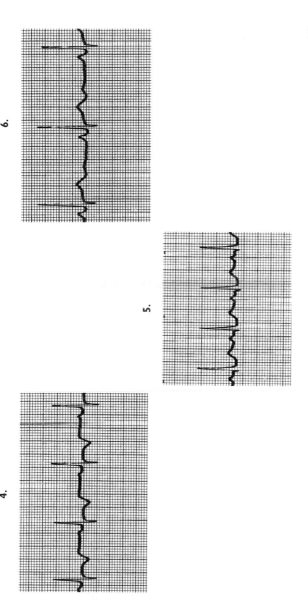

4.

5.

6.

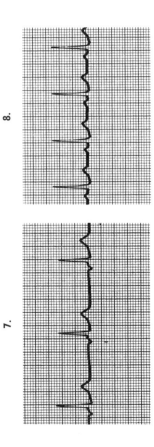

7.

8.

Unit II

Fundamental Techniques of Determining Heart Rate and Rhythm and Performing an ECG

Chapter 4
Estimating Heart Rhythm and Rate From an ECG Strip

Chapter 5
Performing a Single Channel and 12-Lead ECG

In the previous unit you reviewed the basic structure and function of the heart and its electrical conduction system. You learned the physical principles underlying the rationale for electrode and lead placements and how to recognize the components of an ECG. You should now be able to distinguish between isoelectric lines, waveforms, segments, intervals, and the core QRS complex. You are now ready for the next step.

In Unit II, you will learn how to analyze a rhythm strip of ECG paper. You will understand the significance of the 1×1 mm and 5×5 mm blocks relative to estimating rhythm regularity and heart rate. The concepts of time/rate and amplitude/voltage are applied to an ECG strip. You will learn how to count blocks, R waves, and intervals. A normal sinus rhythm will be presented as a baseline from which abnormal rhythms (arrhythmias) will be compared in Units III, IV, and V.

In this unit you will also learn the basic skill of performing an ECG, from equipment assembly, to patient preparation, to appropriate documentation. The procedures for a single channel and multichannel machine are explained.

CHAPTER FOUR

ESTIMATING HEART RHYTHM AND RATE FROM AN ECG STRIP

In the previous three chapters you reviewed the heart's anatomy and physiology and learned the basic components of an ECG. In this chapter you will learn the concepts of time and voltage, how to distinguish between a regular and an irregular rhythm, and how to calculate the heart rate. These concepts are built on an understanding of the rationale behind the construction of the lines and blocks of the ECG paper. Therefore, this chapter begins with a description of the ECG paper.

The ECG Paper

The ECG graph paper is supplied in continuous rolls or packs. The paper has evenly spaced vertical lines (read top to bottom or bottom to top) and horizontal lines (read left to right or right to left) that intersect to form small square blocks and large square blocks. The *horizontal* lines *measure time* in seconds. The *vertical* lines *measure voltage* (*height*) in millimeters (mm). As a frame of reference, 1 inch equals 25 mm. The electrical activities of the heart that occur during polarization, depolarization, and repolarization are transmitted through the ECG electrodes and recorded on special

ECG graph paper. This paper is pressure and heat sensitive. The stylus, a needle-like projection in the recording apparatus of the ECG machine, is heated and transfers the electrical impulses to the graph paper.

REMEMBER

Never fold ECG paper. The strips should always be rolled or looped because they are heat and pressure sensitive. Never touch the heat-sensitive stylus.

The graph paper is designed so that 25 of the 1×1 mm blocks are placed side by side and top to bottom to form a larger square block that equals 5×5 mm. This larger square block is outlined by a line that is darker than the lighter lines shaping the smaller 1×1 mm squares. This basic unit is the building block for interpreting the electrical activity of the heart. When multiple squares are placed side by side, you have your standard strip of ECG graph paper (Fig. 4-1).

Time and Voltage

To interpret the tracings on a strip of ECG paper, you must understand how time and voltage are measured.

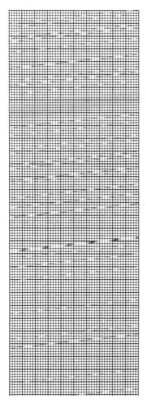

Figure 4-1. A strip of standard ECG paper. Large 5 × 5 mm squares enclosing smaller squares.

Time or Rate

Time or rate is estimated by measuring the number of square blocks *along the horizontal line*. The measurement of *seconds* is used to determine time or rate. The distance across each small square block is 0.04 second (4 hundredths of a second). The distance across one large square block (equal to 5 small blocks) is 5 times greater or 0.2 second (2 tenths of a second). This calculation is reached by multiplying: 0.04 second × 5 squares = 0.2 second. The distance across 5 large square blocks is equal to 1 second. This calculation is reached by multiplying 0.2 second × 5 = 1.0 second (Fig. 4-2).

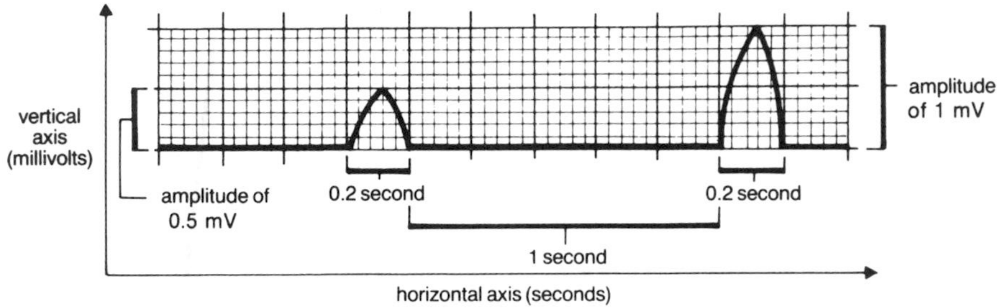

Figure 4-2. Time and voltage measurements on ECG paper.

Amplitude or Voltage

Amplitude or voltage (height or intensity of the electrical impulse) is estimated by measuring the number of square blocks *up or down the vertical line*. The determination of millivolts (mV) estimates the direction and magnitude of the electrical impulse. The voltage of each small square block represents 0.1 mV. The voltage of each large square block (equal to 5 small square blocks) is 5 times greater, or 0.5 mV. This calculation is reached by multiplying 0.1 mV × 5 square blocks = 0.5 mV. Both the horizontal line that measures time and the vertical line that measures voltage are illustrated in Figure 4-2.

Determining Rhythm from the ECG

The term *rhythm* refers to the regularity of a pattern, which in this case is the regularity of the cardiac cycle illustrated by a tracing along a strip of ECG paper. To determine a pattern or rhythm, it is necessary to measure the distance between two complexes and compare this measurement to the next grouping of complexes. This determination is done by measuring the distance from one P wave to the next P wave (atrial activity) or from one R wave to the next R wave (ventricular activity).

If the PP and RR intervals are consistent, then the rhythm is normal or regular; if these interval measurements are not consistent, then the rhythm is abnormal or irregular. A *normal sinus rhythm* occurs when the SA node fires regularly and consistently at a rate of 60 to 100 beats/min. A deviation in rate with a regular rhythm constitutes an arrhythmia. Various types of arrhythmias are presented beginning in Chapter 6.

Normal Sinus Rhythm

Normal sinus rhythm is a regular pattern of heart beats (60–100 beats/min) that repeat every 5 large blocks. Normal P waves precede each QRS complex. The duration of the PR interval and the QRS complex are within normal range. Figure 4-3 is an example of a normal rhythm strip at 82 beats/min.

When the rhythm is regular, measurements can be easily done by just counting the number of large blocks from one P wave to the next P wave or from one R wave to the next R wave (Figs. 4-4 and 4-5). This technique of measuring rhythm regularity should be done across an entire 6-second rhythm strip. The ECG graph paper has small, vertical lines on its upper border marking off 3-second intervals.

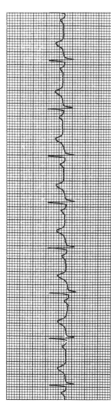

Figure 4-3. Normal sinus rhythm at 82 beats/min.

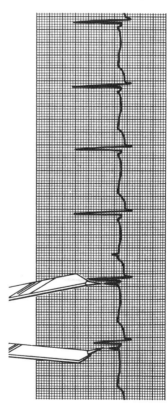

Figure 4-4. Measuring P to P intervals.

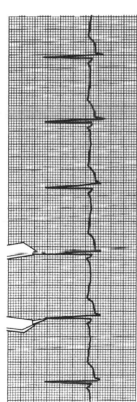

Figure 4-5. Measuring R to R intervals.

Determining Heart Rate

Heart rate is defined as the number of heartbeats that occur *over 1 minute*. Several formulas are used for determining heart rate. A quick formula is shown in Chart 4–1.

Chart 4-1. QUICK FORMULA FOR ESTIMATING HEART RATE

Large Squares Between R Waves that Fall on or Close to Dark Lines	Approximate Heart Rate Per Minute
1	300
2	150
3	100
4	75
5	60
6	50

Regular Pattern or Rhythm

USE THE RR INTERVAL

Estimate Time. Estimate the time in seconds between two R waves (each large square block equals 0.2 second and 5 blocks equal 1 second). Since there are 60 seconds in 1 minute, divide 60 by that number. The number you get is the heart rate. For example, look at Figure 4-6. The duration between the two R waves is 0.88 second. If 60 is divided by 0.88, the heart rate is 68 beats/min.

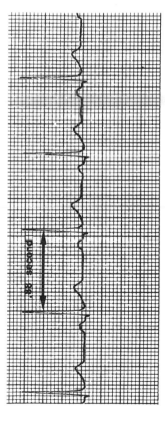

.88 second

60 divided by .88 second = 68 beats / min

Figure 4-6. Estimating time and heart rate using the RR interval.

REMEMBER

When the rhythm is irregular, run a 1-minute strip and count each complex.

Count the R Waves in a 6-Second Strip. Since the ECG graph paper is marked at its upper border with straight vertical lines every 3 seconds, you can count the number of R waves in a 6-second strip. Multiply that number by 10 to find the heart rate in 60 seconds or 1 minute. For example, look at Figure 4-7. There are four RR intervals between two, 3-second increments. Therefore there are $4 \times 10 = 40$ beats/min. The heart rate in this strip is 43 beats/min.

Count the Large Blocks Between R Waves. Begin by finding an R wave that falls on or close to a dark black line. Use that dark line as your starting point to begin counting. Count the number of large blocks, outlined by dark lines, between the two R waves. Use the following formula.

- One large square block between two R waves equals 300 large blocks in a 1-minute strip of ECG paper (heart rate = 300 beats/min).
- Two large blocks between two R waves equals 150 large blocks in a 1-minute strip (heart rate = 150 beats/min).

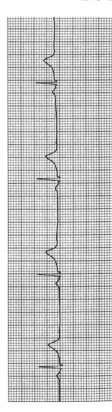

Figure 4-7. Estimating heart rate by counting the R waves. Heart rate is about 43 beats/min.

- A three-block distance equals a heart rate of 100.
- A four-block distance equals a heart rate of 75.
- A five-block distance equals a heart rate of 60.
- A six-block distance equals a heart rate of 50.

When the R waves consistently fall *between* the dark black lines of the large blocks, you can still determine the heart rate by using this formula. You can also simply divide 300 by the exact number of large blocks between the R waves. Figure 4-8 is an example of R waves that fall on a dark line.

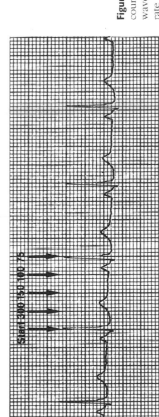

Figure 4-8. Estimating heart rate by counting large blocks between R waves that *fall on dark lines*. Heart rate is about 75 beats/min.

The heart rate is about 75 beats/min. Figure 4-9 is an example of R waves that fall between the dark lines. The heart rate is about 120 beats/min.

An Irregular Pattern or Rhythm

Use these two methods for determining heart rate for an irregular rhythm.

Count the RR Intervals. Count the RR intervals in a 6-second strip (the ECG paper is marked in 3-second increments, equal to 15 large boxes). Multiply that number by 10. Figure 4-10 presents an example of estimating heart rate by counting the RR intervals in a 6-second strip.

Count Each Complex. Another easy yet tedious method is to run a 1-minute strip and count each complex.

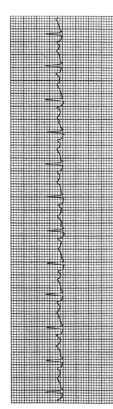

Figure 4-9. Estimating heart rate by counting large blocks between R waves that *fall between the dark lines.* Heart rate is about 120 beats/min.

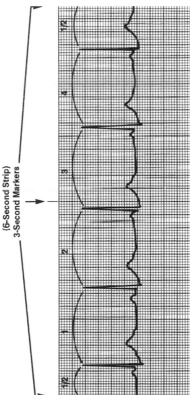

Figure 4-10. Counting RR intervals in a 6-second strip. Heart rate is about 50 beats/min.

63

Analyzing a Rhythm Strip

You now need to practice the basic steps reviewed in this chapter so you can become competent in these skills. The steps for analyzing any rhythm strip have been summarized in Chart 4-2.

Practice Analysis of Rhythm Strips

Examine each of the following eight sample ECG strips. For each, determine whether the rhythm is regular or irregular, calculate the heart rate, examine the P waves, and measure the PR interval and the QRS complex. Describe your interpretation of the rhythm. Write your answers on the lines provided.

Chart 4-2. Analyzing a Rhythm Strip: A Standard 10-Step Process

1. *Determine the rhythm.* Is it regular, abnormal, or irregular?
2. *Determine the rate.* Is it normal, fast or slow?
3. *Count the rate.*
4. *Find the P wave.* Does it precede each QRS complex? If absent, what waveform replaces it? Is it similar in configuration?
5. *Measure the PR interval.* Count the squares from the beginning of the P wave to the beginning of the QRS complex. Multiply by 0.04 second. The normal range is 0.12 to 0.20 second. Accelerated or shortened PR intervals may be indicative of myocardial disease and/or conduction abnormalities.
6. *Examine the Q waves.* Are they pathologic? Are they greater than 3 mm in height and/or greater than 1/3 the height of the R wave?

7. *Measure the QRS complex.* Count the number of squares from the beginning of the QRS to its end. Multiply by 0.04 second. Are they similar in configuration? Do they vary in composition? The normal range is 0.04–0.10 second.
8. *Examine the ST segments.* Normal elevation or depression is 1 mm. Deviations occur in ischemia and myocardial infarction.
9. *Check the T waves.* T waves should be upright in all leads except leads III, aVR and V_1. Check for positive or negative deflections or inversion.
10. *Measure the QT interval.* Is it shortened or prolonged? The normal range is 0.32 to 0.40 second. It should be less than 1/2 the distance of the preceding RR interval. Prolonged or shortened intervals may indicate pharmacologic effects or electrolyte abnormalities; ie, hypocalcemia, class I antiarrhythmics, or tricyclic antidepressants.

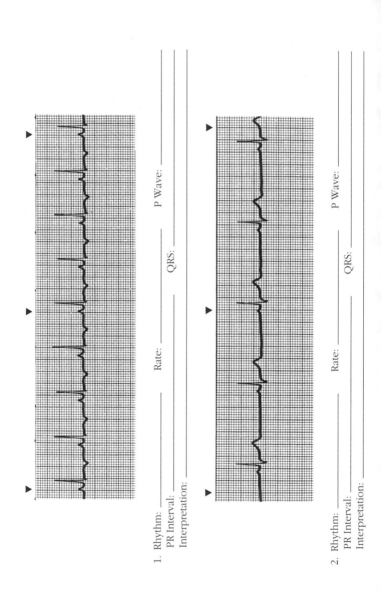

1. Rhythm: _____   Rate: _____   P Wave: _____
   PR Interval: _____   QRS: _____
   Interpretation: _____

2. Rhythm: _____   Rate: _____   P Wave: _____
   PR Interval: _____   QRS: _____
   Interpretation: _____

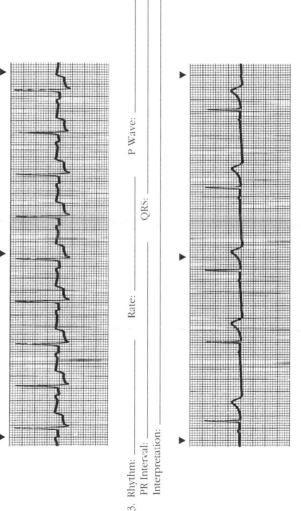

3. Rhythm: _____   Rate: _____   P Wave: _____

   PR Interval: _____   QRS: _____

   Interpretation: _____

4. Rhythm: _____   Rate: _____   P Wave: _____

   PR Interval: _____   QRS: _____

   Interpretation: _____

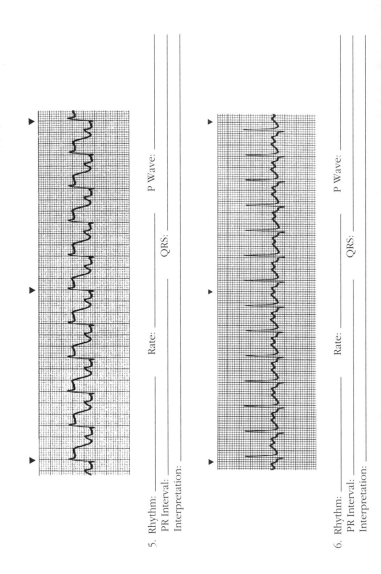

5. Rhythm: _____ Rate: _____ P Wave: _____
   PR Interval: _____ QRS: _____
   Interpretation: _____

6. Rhythm: _____ Rate: _____ P Wave: _____
   PR Interval: _____ QRS: _____
   Interpretation: _____

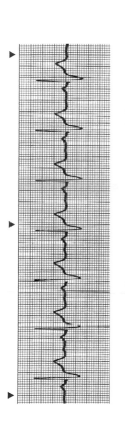

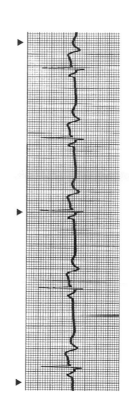

7. Rhythm: _____   Rate: _____   P Wave: _____
   PR Interval: _____   QRS: _____
   Interpretation: _____

8. Rhythm: _____   Rate: _____   P Wave: _____
   PR Interval: _____   QRS: _____
   Interpretation: _____

CHAPTER FIVE

PERFORMING A SINGLE CHANNEL AND 12-LEAD ECG

You should now have a basic understanding about the electrical conductivity of the heart, be able to recognize normal sinus rhythm, and calculate heart rate from an ECG strip. Now you will learn how to prepare your patient for this noninvasive procedure. The steps for performing an ECG on an adult are outlined below. Pediatric considerations are included throughout.

Preparing for the ECG

Before beginning, check the physician's order for the ECG and note any comments about the patient that may influence either the procedure or the patient's reaction to the test. For example, document any medications the patient may be taking.

ASSEMBLE EQUIPMENT

- Collect the ECG machine.
- Obtain the disposable, pregelled electrodes.

- Obtain a roll of ECG paper.
- Collect sterile wipes or 2 × 2 inch gauze and alcohol.
- Gather a safety razor and shaving cream to remove thick hair from areas of the skin where the electrodes will be placed. If the patient is taking an anticoagulant, such as Coumadin, an electric razor is recommended.

CHECK EQUIPMENT

- Plug in the machine. Make sure it is working.
- Check that enough paper is loaded into the machine, and if necessary, load additional ECG paper.
- Make sure the standardization is set. All machines have a standardization mechanism (a button labeled "STD") that can be set to be consistent with an internationally accepted code.
- *Note:* Use a battery-powered ECG machine for patients with external pacing wires unless otherwise ordered by a physician.

PREPARE THE PATIENT

- If the patient is a child, you may need a parent or a staff person to assist you.
- Introduce yourself to the patient.
- Check for patient identification.
- Explain the procedure; verify that the patient understands.
- Explain that the procedure is painless, that there are no risks, and that the electrodes do not emit electricity.

- For a child, make sure you use words that are easy to understand. Name the body part that will be touched; use exact words, not abstract terms. A young child may be afraid of being "shocked." Expect crying from a child.
- Provide for patient privacy.
- Wash your hands.
- Ask or assist the patient to undress, making sure the wrists, chest, and ankles are without clothing. Cover the patient's chest with a towel or drape to maintain privacy. Nylon stockings may be left in place. A patient gown may be worn.
- For a child, restraints may be necessary. Sometimes a helpful parent can encourage a child to remain still and quiet.
- Ask the patient to lie down in bed; assist a child.
- Make sure all jewelry is removed.
- Cleanse the skin area thoroughly to remove oil, dirt, and perspiration. Clean an area larger than you need for electrode placement. Dry skin thoroughly.
- Make sure the patient is comfortable and able to relax the legs and arms. It is sometimes helpful to raise the head of the bed.
- Open the sealed package containing the disposable silver/silver chloride electrodes. Most electrodes are pregelled, adhesive, and attached to a backing material (usually foam) that is peeled away before use. Some electrodes require the application of a water-soluble gel or another conductive material (Fig. 5-1).

Place the electrode sticky side down on the cleansed area, starting in on corner. Avoid touching the sticky side.

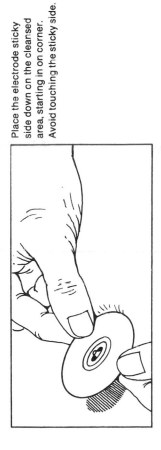

Smooth the electrode on the skin in a circular motion. Make sure the saline pad is in good contact with the skin. Connect the monitor wire to the center of the electrode.

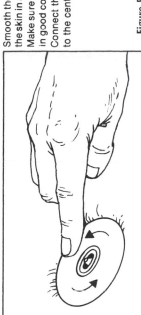

Figure 5-1. Application of electrode leads.

- Peel each electrode from its backing material and *firmly* place the electrodes on the fleshiest portion of the upper arms and lower legs. Make sure each pad has good skin contact. If you are using suction cup electrodes, apply conductive gel to the cup and on the metal electrode plate.

- Apply limb leads, which are color coded, accordingly:
  - Right arm—white
  - Left arm—black
  - Right leg—green
  - Left leg—red

- Apply the six chest (V) leads, as follows:
  - V_1—fourth intercostal space, right of sternum
  - V_2—fourth intercostal space, left of sternum
  - V_3—diagonally between V_2 and V_4, left midclavicular line
  - V_4—fifth intercostal space, left midclavicular line
  - V_5—fifth intercostal space, between V_4 and V_6, left anterior axillary line, below the armpit
  - V_6—fifth intercostal space, left, midaxillary line

- Advise the patient to lie still, relax, breathe normally, and avoid talking and coughing while the ECG is recording.

Additionally, leads may be applied to enhance the analysis of the patient's cardiac status. This may be seen in patients with suspected right ventricular infarct, dextrocardia, or right axis deviation. Since neonates typically have a right axis deviation, it is common to perform a 15-lead ECG, which includes the standard leads along with V_3R, V_4R and V_7. When more detailed analysis of the posterior wall of the heart needs to be performed, as in a posterior MI, leads V_7 and V_8 are used. An 18-lead ECG would include all of the following:

- Right precordial leads
  - V_3R—diagonally between V_1 and V_4R
  - V_4R—fifth intercostal space, right midclavicular line
  - V_5R—fifth intercostal space, right anterior axillary line
  - V_6R—fifth intercostal space, right midaxillary line
- Posterior leads
  - V_7—fifth intercostal space, left posterior axillary line
  - V_8—fifth intercostal space, left posterior midscapular line

Recording the ECG

Single Channel Machine

Older, single channel machines require manually performing those functions that newer machines automatically perform. One lead is recorded at a time and you will have to turn the dial manually for each lead you are recording and manually move each lead to every "V" position.

- Make sure that the ECG machine is plugged in and grounded. Review manufacturer's directions.
- Set the lead selector switch to STD. Set the standardization (the standard running speed is 25 mm/s).

- Turn the recorder switch to RUN.
- Center the baseline by using the position control knob.
- Make certain that the standardization is set at 10 mm.
- Turn lead selector switch to lead I. Run 8 to 10 inches of tracing and label.
- Complete for the remaining leads, labeling each lead.
- Turn the machine to "pause."
- Position the chest electrodes for V₁.
- Turn the selector switch to STD and the recorder switch to RUN, and insert the standardization.
- Turn the selector switch to V and the recorder switch to ON and run 5 to 6 inches of tracing.
- Label lead and turn recorder switch off.
- Move chest electrode to next position and repeat previous steps for the remaining chest leads.
- Turn the lead selector switch to STD slowly and run until baseline appears.
- Turn the recorder switch off and unplug the machine.
- Label the ECG strip with the patient's name, room and bed number, date, and time.
- Be careful not to show alarm or concern if you notice an arrhythmia because this may upset the patient.
- Take the ECG recording to the appropriate person or place it in the patient's chart or medical record.

Multichannel Machine

- Enter the patient's identification information into the machine. This will be printed on the ECG paper.
- Push a button, usually marked "AUTO" to begin recording. This machine automatically records all the leads at one time or a rhythm strip (limb leads) as requested by the physician.
- Observe recording as the strip is running. Make sure that all leads are graphed.
- Check for any artifacts that may be caused by something you can correct (ie, loose electrodes). For a child, make sure movements do not cause artifacts that may be misinterpreted.
- Be careful not to show alarm or concern if you notice an arrhythmia because your facial expressions or behavior may upset the patient. Consistently comfort a child throughout the procedure.

Completing the Procedure

PERFORM FINAL STEPS

- Turn off the machine and obtain the recorded strip.
- Remove the electrodes from the patient.
- Clean the skin and wipe off any excess gel or paste.
- Help the patient to put gown back on. It may be necessary to dress the child, especially if child is upset. Frequently a parent assumes this responsibility.
- Comfort as necessary because the patient may be concerned about his or her medical condition.

- Apply covers or blankets as necessary to provide warmth and privacy.
- Thank the patient and say good-bye.

DOCUMENT APPROPRIATELY

- Take ECG recording to the appropriate person or place in the patient's chart or medical record.

MAINTAIN THE EQUIPMENT

- Clean the machine according to agency policy.
- Restock electrode patches, conductive gel, and so forth.
- Secure the electrical cord and lead wires so damage does not occur in transport.
- Store or transport machine as necessary.

Unit Summary

You have now learned all the basic foundation concepts and skills necessary to perform an ECG, identify a normal rhythm strip, and calculate heart rate. You should be comfortable enough to move forward to the next level of recognizing and interpreting arrhythmias. The next unit discusses arrhythmias of a sinus and atrial origin.

Arrhythmias of Sinus and Atrial Origin

In Units I and II you learned the basics of the ECG. You reviewed the anatomy and electrical conduction of the heart, learned how to record an ECG, how to calculate rate and rhythm, how deflections are formed from electrical activity, and how the various components of the ECG (waveforms, intervals, etc) reflect electrical conduction.

In Unit III you will learn how to read an ECG strip and recognize the most common sinus and atrial arrhythmias, and those AV junctional arrhythmias and blocks that you may encounter in your practice. You are not expected to become an expert in reading ECGs. However, you will be held accountable for recognizing common patterns, identifying potentially life-threatening arrhythmias, and communicating relevant information quickly to the appropriate professional staff person.

An *arrhythmia* is any disturbance in the rate, rhythm, origin, or conduction of the cardiac electrical impulse. Not every arrhythmia is dangerous, but most require medical intervention, hospitalization, or long-term management. Unfortunately some arrhythmias cause sudden death. Arrhythmias are divided into four basic categories: sinus node disturbances, conduction blocks, ectopic beats, and preexcitation syndromes.

Arrhythmias result from a variety of disorders and precipitating factors. Respiratory causes include pulmonary disorders and chronic lung disease that result in decreased oxygenation to the myocardium. Electrolyte disturbances and medications, especially drugs used for long-term management of chronic illnesses, can increase sympathetic tone and cause irritability and arrhythmias. Cardiac causes include cardiac cell irritability secondary to cellular ischemia (angina pectoris) and injury (MI).

A major source of arrhythmias is enlargement and hypertrophy of the atria and ventricles, most significantly, left ventricular hypertrophy. CHF and valvular heart disease also cause severe arrhythmias that can result in death.

The next three chapters address arrhythmias of various origins. In Chapter 6, arrhythmias of sinus origin are divided into five basic categories: sinus bradycardia, sinus tachycardia, sinus arrhythmia, sinus exit block, and sinus arrest. Atrial arrhythmias in Chapter 7 are divided into five basic categories: wandering pacemaker, premature atrial contractions, paroxysmal atrial tachycardia, atrial flutter, and atrial fibrillation. In Chapter 8, AV junctional arrhythmias are divided into four categories: premature junctional contractions, paroxysmal junctional tachycardia, AV junctional escape beats, and junctional escape rhythms. AV blocks are divided according to the degree of blockage, creating the categories of first-, second-, and third-degree AV blocks.

It is important that you learn how to recognize these common arrhythmias and identify potentially lethal ECG patterns. To facilitate this process, each arrhythmia is explained and outlined according to etiology, symptomatology, primary treatment goals, and specific arrhythmia characteristics. A sample ECG pattern is provided for each arrhythmia to illustrate the outlined description. Arrhythmia strips are also included for practice exercises. Good luck as you begin your new journey!

CHAPTER SIX
ARRHYTHMIAS OF SINUS ORIGIN

The origin of a normal heart rhythm is the SA node in the right atrium. This SA node is a reliable pacemaker that is affected by such things as the autonomic nervous system, hormones, medications, illness, and especially diseases of a cardiac or pulmonary nature. The five sinus arrhythmias you should be able to identify after you complete this chapter are sinus bradycardia, sinus tachycardia, sinus arrhythmia, sinus exit block, and sinus arrest. Each is presented briefly along with abbreviated information about etiology, symptomatology, treatment modalities, and defining characteristics.

REMEMBER

✓ Your role, as a health care practitioner, is to recognize deviations, identify arrhythmia patterns to the best of your ability, and communicate relevant information to the appropriate health care professional.

Normal Sinus Rhythm

Normal sinus rhythm occurs when the SA node fires regularly and consistently at the rate of 60 to 100 beats/min. Normal P waves precede each QRS complex. The duration of the PR interval and the QRS complex are within normal range. A more detailed explanation of normal sinus rhythm was originally presented in Chapter 4. Refer back to that chapter for review if necessary.

Sinus Bradycardia

Sinus bradycardia is an SA node arrhythmia that exhibits a normal rhythm pattern except that the heart rate is below 60 beats/min. The ECG pattern repeats itself at intervals of greater duration than every 5 large blocks. Impulses follow the normal pathway through the conduction system. P waves and QRS complexes are normal in duration and pattern. In some individuals and athletes, a rate of less than 60 beats/min is normal.

ETIOLOGY

- Increased vagal stimulation
- Medical conditions: anorexia nervosa, atherosclerotic heart disease, hypoendocrine states (ie, Addison's disease, myxedema), hypothermia, increased intracranial pressure, MI

- Medications: antihypertensives, β blockers, calcium channel blockers, CNS depressants (ie, morphine, sedatives), digoxin (especially digitalis toxicity)
- Normal variation of heart rate occurs in athletes and healthy young adults.

SYMPTOMS

In general, the symptoms seen with sinus bradycardia are all related to decreased cardiac output.
- Cardiac: chest pressure and pain, dyspnea, hypotension
- Neurologic: dizziness, seizures, syncope

PRIMARY TREATMENT GOALS

- Insertion or application of a pacemaker may be indicated.
- Management and elimination of the cause of bradycardia
- Medications: IV atropine may be required
- Stimulation of the sympathetic nervous system
- Suppression of the parasympathetic nervous system
- Treatment may not be necessary if the patient is asymptomatic.

ARRHYTHMIA CHARACTERISTICS

- Rate: 40 to 60 beats/min
- Rhythm: regular to slightly irregular
- Conduction: usually normal

- P waves: one P wave precedes each QRS complex
- PR interval: within normal range (0.12–0.20 second)
- QRS complex: usually normal (0.06–0.12 second) and consistent in shape

SAMPLE ECG STRIP

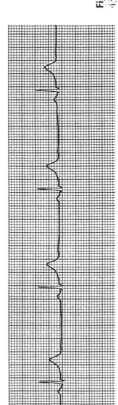

Figure 6-1. Sinus bradycardia at 43 beats/min.

Sinus Tachycardia

Sinus tachycardia is one of the most common SA node arrhythmias that exhibit a normal rhythm pattern with a heart rate that is faster than 100 beats/min. The ECG pattern repeats itself at intervals less than every 3 large blocks. Impulses follow the normal pathway through the conduction system.

ETIOLOGY

- Diet: caffeine-containing beverages (coffee, soda, tea) and chocolate
- Life-style: smoking and use of nicotine
- Medical conditions may include but are not limited to aremia, anxiety, fever, hemorrhage, hypotension, pain, and shock.
- Medications: CNS stimulants (dopamine, epinephrine)
- Myocardial damage from infection, injury, or trauma

SYMPTOMS

The primary symptoms of tachycardia are related to decreased cardiac output.

- Cardiac: chest pressure and pain, decreased diastolic refilling, dyspnea, and a characteristic "fluttering" in the chest. The major concern with tachycardia is that, as the rate increases (serious symptoms are seen at a rate > 160 beats/min), over days or weeks, diastolic refilling is diminished and cardiac output is decreased. Eventually heart failure may occur.
- Neurologic: dizziness, syncope

PRIMARY TREATMENT GOALS

- Application of carotid sinus pressure as a temporary measure for a rapid heart rate that is resistant to returning to a normal range
- Cardiac drugs: calcium channel blockers, digoxin, and propranolol (Inderal)
- Elimination of the cause of the tachycardia

- Use of minor tranquilizers or antianxiety agents to depress the CNS

ARRHYTHMIA CHARACTERISTICS

- Rate: greater than 100 beats/min; can range up to 180 beats/min
- Rhythm: regular
- Conduction: usually normal
- P waves: one P wave precedes each QRS complex but may be buried in a preceding T wave
- PR interval: within normal range
- QRS complex: usually normal

SAMPLE ECG STRIP

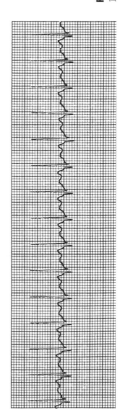

Figure 6-2. Sinus tachycardia at 149 beats/min.

Sinus Arrhythmia

This arrhythmia occurs when an electrical impulse at the SA node is discharged at a normal rate but at an irregular interval.

ETIOLOGY

The most common cause is the normal variation in pressure within the chest during inspiration and expiration, with inspiration accelerating the heart rate and expiration slowing the heart rate. Sinus arrhythmia is common in young adults who have a slower than normal heart rate.

SYMPTOMS

This condition is usually asymptomatic, with a small possibility of decreased cardiac output.

PRIMARY TREATMENT GOALS

No treatment is necessary unless cardiac output is compromised.

ARRHYTHMIA CHARACTERISTICS

- Rate: usually 60 to 100 beats/min; can be slower or faster
- Rhythm: irregular with corresponding changes in the rate
- Conduction: usually normal
- P waves: one P wave precedes each QRS complex

- PR interval: within normal range
- QRS complex: usually normal

SAMPLE ECG STRIP

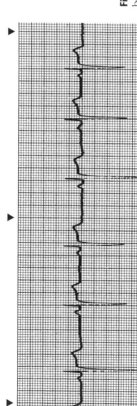

Figure 6-3. Sinus arrhythmia at 60 beats/min.

Sinus Exit Block

This arrhythmia occurs when normally discharged atrial impulses are blocked within the SA node (Fig. 6-4). The pattern is easily recognized by missing beats in the cardiac cycle, after which the rhythm returns in cadence, at a time that is an exact multiple of the previous RR or PP interval.

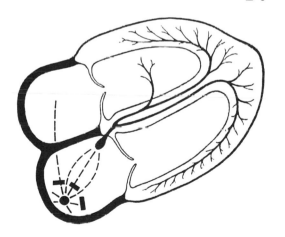

Figure 6-4. Cardiac illustration of sinus exit block.

ETIOLOGY

- Cardiac disease: CAD, CHF, MI
- Increased vagal stimulation
- Medications: digitalis, procainamide, quinidine

SYMPTOMS

Symptoms are not significant if block is intermittent; symptoms do not usually last longer than 3 seconds.

- Cardiac: palpitations (infrequent blocks)
- Neurologic: dizziness, syncope (prolonged blocks)

PRIMARY TREATMENT GOALS

No treatment is required if the patient is asymptomatic.

- Management protocol is similar to that for bradycardia.
- Medications: IV atropine sulfate if aggressive measures are needed

ARRHYTHMIA CHARACTERISTICS

- Rate: usually less than 60 beats/min because of missed beats; can be normal
- Rhythm: irregular pattern characterized by missed beats followed by a return of rhythm in cadence. Pattern is usually regular before and after the missed beats.
- Conduction: usually normal

- P wave: one P wave precedes each QRS complex; will be absent during missed beats
- PR interval: absent during pause
- QRS complex: usually normal, will be absent during missed beats

SAMPLE ECG STRIP

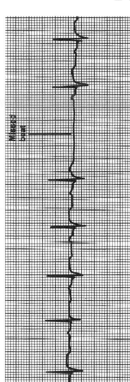

Figure 6-5. Sinus exit block reflecting a missed beat.

Sinus Arrest

This arrhythmia occurs when the SA node stops discharging impulses and alternate pacemaker cells take over.

ETIOLOGY

- Cardiac disease is the most severe cause: cardiomyopathy, rheumatic heart disease, MI
- Similar to sinus bradycardia and sinus block

SYMPTOMS

Symptoms are usually of shortened duration (< 3 seconds).

- Cardiac: dyspnea
- Neurologic: dizziness, syncope

PRIMARY TREATMENT GOALS

- Insert permanent pacemaker if necessary
- Medications: atropine sulfate, epinephrine
- Prevent the progression of arrhythmia into asystole
- Reduce or eliminate any medications that may be contributing to the cause

ARRHYTHMIA CHARACTERISTICS

- Rate: usually less than 60 beats/min because of missed beats
- Rhythm: irregular patterns characterized by missed beats; regular rhythm returns before and after pause
- Conduction: usually normal
- P wave: one P wave precedes each QRS complex; will be absent during missed beats

- PR interval: absent during pause
- QRS complex: usually normal; will be absent during missed beats

SAMPLE ECG STRIP

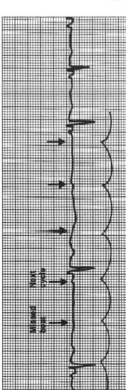

Missed beat

Next cycle

Figure 6-6. Sinus arrest reflecting missed beats.

Practice Rhythm Strip Analysis

Examine each of the following 10 sample sinus arrhythmias. Identify each arrhythmia and describe significant characteristics Write your answers on the lines provided.

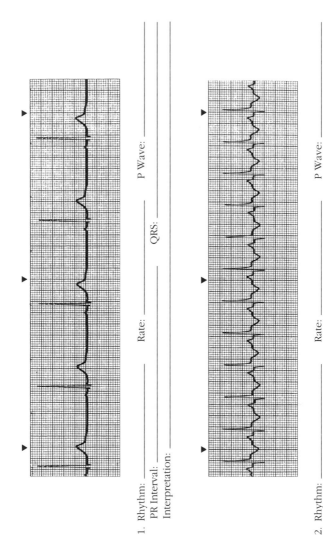

1. Rhythm: _____   Rate: _____   P Wave: _____

   PR Interval: _____   QRS: _____

   Interpretation: _____

2. Rhythm: _____   Rate: _____   P Wave: _____

   PR Interval: _____   QRS: _____

   Interpretation: _____

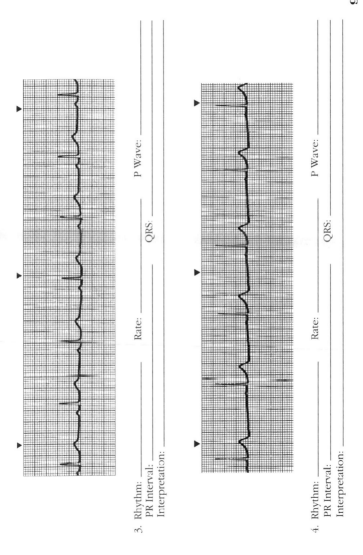

3. Rhythm: _____ Rate: _____ P Wave: _____
   PR Interval: _____ QRS: _____
   Interpretation: _____

4. Rhythm: _____ Rate: _____ P Wave: _____
   PR Interval: _____ QRS: _____
   Interpretation: _____

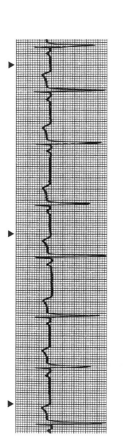

5. Rhythm: _____ Rate: _____ P Wave: _____
   PR Interval: _____ QRS: _____
   Interpretation: _____

6. Rhythm: _____ Rate: _____ P Wave: _____
   PR Interval: _____ QRS: _____
   Interpretation: _____

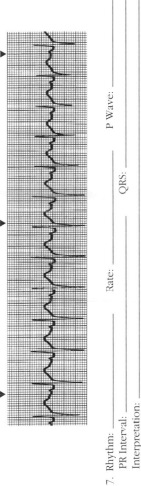

▶

7. Rhythm: _____ Rate: _____ P Wave: _____

   PR Interval: _____ QRS: _____

   Interpretation: _____

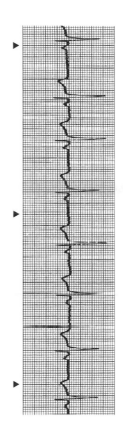

▶

8. Rhythm: _____ Rate: _____ P Wave: _____

   PR Interval: _____ QRS: _____

   Interpretation: _____

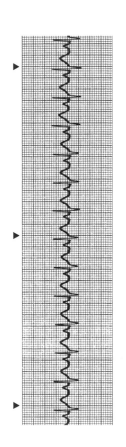

9. Rhythm: _____ Rate: _____ P Wave: _____
   PR Interval: _____ QRS: _____
   Interpretation: _____

10. Rhythm: _____ Rate: _____ P Wave: _____
    PR Interval: _____ QRS: _____
    Interpretation: _____

CHAPTER SEVEN
ATRIAL ARRHYTHMIAS

The SA node, the pacemaker of the heart, initiates the cardiac impulse that depolarizes the remainder of the heart. If the SA node fails to discharge, other pacemakers are stimulated to depolarize, the atria being the first to respond with a rate similar or more rapid than the inherent rate of the SA node. The electrical impulses that originate from irritable tissue (foci) outside the SA node are called *ectopic beats*.

Atrial impulses originating outside the SA node are evident on the ECG by the appearance of abnormally shaped P waves. The rapidity of the beat changes the appearance of the P wave from pointed to sawtoothed and then to wavy. As the rate increases, ventricular filling is compromised, which in turn diminishes cardiac output. After you complete this chapter, you should be able to identify five atrial arrhythmias: wandering atrial pacemaker, premature atrial contractions, paroxysmal atrial tachycardia, atrial flutter, and atrial fibrillation.

Wandering Pacemaker

A wandering pacemaker occurs when the pacemaker site generating the ectopic beat switches from one location to another, usually at a site between the SA node, the AV junction, and other sites within the atrium. A wandering pacemaker can be found in young adults, especially athletes. It usually carries no inherent risk.

A distinguishing characteristic is the regularity of the rhythm as the pacemaker site changes (Fig. 7-1). The appearance of the P wave (upright, peaked, flat, or inverted) helps establish pacemaker origin. Ventricular contractions are usually not affected because the impulse follows the normal conduction pathway after passing through the AV node. An accurate diagnosis depends on the identification of three differently shaped P waves in a strip.

ETIOLOGY

- Cardiac disease: cardiac ischemia, CAD, CHF, MI
- Increased vagal stimulation
- May be nonspecific
- Medications: digitalis

SYMPTOMS

Symptoms may not be present and the rhythm disturbance may resolve itself.

PRIMARY TREATMENT GOALS

- Treatment may not be necessary if patient is asymptomatic.
- Discontinue medications that may be causing the symptoms.

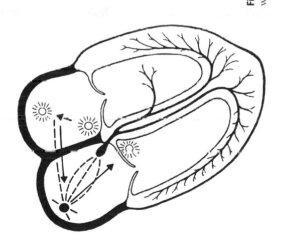

Figure 7-1. Cardiac illustration of a wandering pacemaker.

ARRHYTHMIA CHARACTERISTICS

- Rate: variable, usually 60 to 100 beats/min
- Rhythm: regular to slightly irregular; pattern depends on pacemaker site
- Conduction: usually normal, depends on site of pacemaker
- P waves: variable in shape, one P wave before each QRS except where pacemaker site is junctional; may be hidden in QRS complex
- PR interval: varies depending on site of pacemaker
- QRS complex: usually normal

SAMPLE ECG STRIP

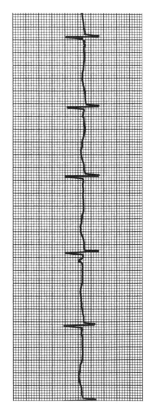

Figure 7-2. A wandering pacemaker.

Premature Atrial Contractions

Premature atrial contractions (PACs), one of the most common ectopic beats, occurs when an impulse is generated by an irritable area of tissue in the atria rather than by the SA node. This ectopic beat interrupts the normal rhythm and is evidenced by abnormally shaped P waves that can be singula-, bigeminal (every other beat), trigeminal (every third beat), or clustered. Three or more PACs are referred to as paroxysmal atrial tachycardia (PAT). Occasionally an *escape atrial beat* will occur late in a cardiac cycle. Similar to a PAC, escape beats require no treatment. The QRS complex should not be affected because ventricular depolarization occurs in a regular pattern.

ETIOLOGY

- Cardiac disease: CHF, MI, atrial enlargement
- Diet: caffeine-containing beverages (coffee, soda, tea)
- Electrolyte disturbances: hypokalemia, hypermetabolic states
- Emotions: anxiety, excitement, fear, stress
- Life-style: exercise, excessive use of alcohol or nicotine
- Medical conditions: chronic obstructive pulmonary disease
- Medications: CNS system stimulants and OTC drugs containing stimulants

SYMPTOMS

- Cardiac: feelings of palpitations or a "skipped beat," possible pulse deficit (difference between apical and radial pulse rate)

PRIMARY TREATMENT GOALS

Treatment may not be required.

- Decrease consumption of beverages with caffeine.
- Decrease stress.
- Medications if PACs are greater than 6 beats/min: antianxiety agents, β blockers, calcium antagonists, digitalis

ARRHYTHMIA CHARACTERISTICS

- Rate: 60 to 100 beats/min, can occur with rates less than 60 or more than 60 beats/min
- Rhythm: regular except when PACs occur. The P wave will occur early in the cycle and will not have a complete compensatory pause (pause during which SA node "resets" and does not fire any impulse).
- Conduction: usually normal; some premature P waves will not be followed by a QRS complex.
- P waves: premature; different configuration than P waves that originate in SA node; may be hidden in the preceding T wave
- PR interval: different from PR intervals created by ectopic foci; can be shorter or longer in duration
- QRS complex: usually normal, may be absent or distorted; complexes may not follow every P wave

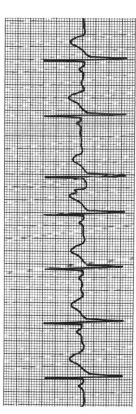

Figure 7-3. Premature atrial contraction.

Paroxysmal Atrial Tachycardia

Paroxysmal atrial tachycardia (PAT) is caused by an irritable area of tissue in the atria that dominates the SA node and takes over the heart's pacemaker function (Fig. 7-4). PATs are frequently preceded by PACs; they usually start abruptly and end just as suddenly. The rapid rate of the arrhythmia (150–250 beats/min), prevents the ventricles from adequately filling, thereby decreasing cardiac output. This is more serious in the elderly and in those with preexisting cardiac disorders.

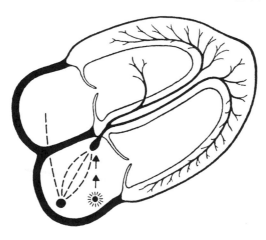

Figure 7-4. Cardiac illustration of paroxysmal atrial tachycardia.

ETIOLOGY

- Not usually associated with organic heart disease
- Same conditions and factors that cause PACs

SYMPTOMS

Symptoms are directly proportional to the cause and the rapidity of the atrial contractions.

- Cardiac: chest pain, dyspnea, hypotension with a small pulse pressure, palpitations, weak rapid pulse
- Neurologic: dizziness, syncope

PRIMARY TREATMENT GOALS

Treatment is directed toward eliminating the cause.

- Cardiac drugs: diltiazem (Cardizem), verapamil, digoxin, propranolol, procainamide (Pronestyl), quinidine, and vasopressors to slow rate
- Cardioversion when other measures do not work
- Carotid sinus pressure, the gag reflex, and the Valsalva maneuver (forceful exhaling with glottis, nose and mouth closed)
- Vagal nerve stimulation to decrease the heart rate

ARRHYTHMIA CHARACTERISTICS

- Rate: 150 to 250 beats/min
- Rhythm: regular to slightly irregular

- Conduction: usually normal
- P waves: ectopic and distorted; may be hidden in preceding T waves or in QRS complexes
- PR interval: less than 0.12 second; usually hidden and not measurable
- QRS complex: usually normal (< 0.12 second); may be distorted

SAMPLE ECG STRIP

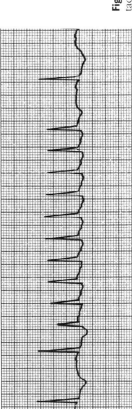

Figure 7-5. Paroxysmal atrial tachycardia.

Atrial Flutter

Atrial flutter is an arrhythmia generated by a rapid, irritable focus in the atria that discharges impulses at the rate of 250 to 400 beats/min (Fig. 7-6). This rate is faster than the ventricles can contract (never > 250 beats/min).

With atrial flutter a unique mechanism occurs whereby the transmission of the rapidly firing impulses is intermittently blocked at the AV node, thus preventing damage to the ventricles. Impulses that pass through may do so in consistent intervals, that is every second beat, every third beat, or every fourth beat, or variable intervals. A consistent block is referred to by the ratio of atrial to ventricular beats (2:1, 3:1, or 4:1).

ETIOLOGY

Atrial flutter is caused by the same conditions that cause PACs.

- Irritable area of atrial tissue
- Medical conditions: usually found in underlying cardiac disease, especially after MI; cardiomyopathy, CHF, and valvular heart disease

SYMPTOMS

- Cardiac: chest pain and pressure, dyspnea, feelings of palpitations, "skipped beats"
- Neurologic: dizziness, syncope

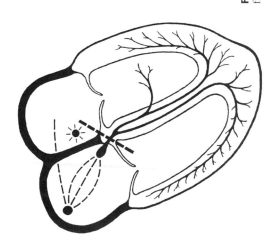

Figure 7-6. Cardiac illustration of atrial flutter.

Primary Treatment Goals

- Cardiac drugs: Cardizem, digoxin, Pronestyl, propranolol, quinidine sulfate, and verapamil hydrochloride to slow the rate and increase the AV node block
- Electrical cardioversion is the initial treatment of choice.

Arrhythmia Characteristics

- Rate
  - Atrial: 250 to 400 beats/min
  - Ventricular: depends on AV blockage; usually 2:1, 3:1, 4:1. Goal is controlled management at less than 100 beats/min.
- Rhythm: regular or irregular, depending on the regularity of the block. For example, if the block varies from 4:1 to 3:1, then the rhythm is irregular. If the block is consistently 3:1, then the rhythm is regular.
- Conduction: depends on rate and AV blockage
- P waves: characteristic sawtooth appearance, peaked or rounded and appearing uniform in shape; sometimes called F waves or flutter waves
- PR interval: not usually measurable
- QRS complex: usually normal; sometimes distorted because P waves alter configuration. T waves are usually hidden or distorted.

111

Sample ECG Strip

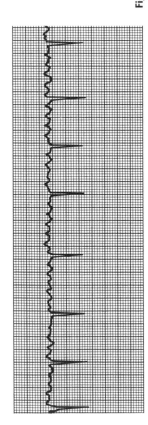

Figure 7-7. Atrial flutter.

Atrial Fibrillation

Atrial fibrillation is caused by multiple irritable foci in the atria leading to a disorganized and unco-ordinated twitching of the atrial musculature (Fig. 7-8). The AV node intermittently blocks the passage of the 350 to 500 impulses/min from passing down to the ventricles. However, rapid ventricular con-tractions do result in diminished ventricular filling and reduced stroke volume, by as much as 20%.

ETIOLOGY

Atrial fibrillation is caused by the same factors that cause PACs and PATs.

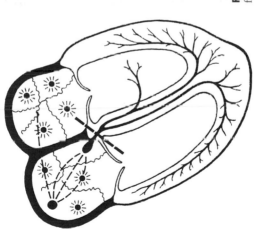

Figure 7-8. Cardiac illustration of atrial fibrillation.

113

- Medical conditions: atherosclerotic heart disease, CAD, chronic obstructive lung disease, MI; also found with valvular heart disease and pulmonary embolism (pooled atrial blood forms thrombi)

SYMPTOMS

- Cardiac: reduced cardiac output by 10% to 25% with associated symptoms—chest pressure and pain, dyspnea, hypotension, pulse deficit, CHF
- Decreased kidney perfusion
- Neurologic: dizziness, syncope
- Pulmonary emboli (because of quivering atria, dormant blood in atria forms clots)

PRIMARY TREATMENT GOALS

Treatment is directed toward decreasing atrial irritability and decreasing ventricular contractions.

- Electrical cardioversion if medications fail
- Medications: anticoagulants to prevent pulmonary emboli, β blockers, calcium antagonists, and digitalis

ARRHYTHMIA CHARACTERISTICS

- Rate
  - Atrial: 350 to 600 beats/min; usually unable to estimate rate because of the rapidity of the beats; no distinct P waves
  - Ventricular: can range from 100 to 250 beats/min depending on impulses sent from atria; goal is controlled management at less than 100 beats/min.

- Rhythm: irregular and very rapid, influenced by degree of AV blockage
- Conduction: ventricles respond irregularly to atrial impulses
- P waves: characterized by twitching, cannot be identified; wavelike deflections cover the baseline
- PR interval: cannot be measured
- QRS complex: usually normal; occasionally distorted due to rapidly firing P waves

SAMPLE ECG STRIP

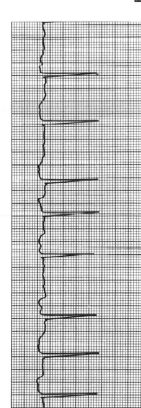

Figure 7-9. Atrial fibrillation.

Practice Rhythm Strip Analysis

Examine each of the following 10 sample atrial arrhythmias. Identify each arrhythmia and describe significant characteristics. Write your answers on the lines provided.

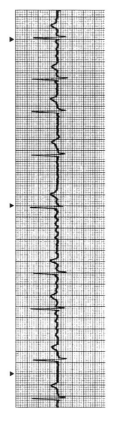
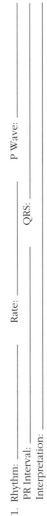

1. Rhythm: _____   Rate: _____   P Wave: _____
   PR Interval: _____   QRS: _____
   Interpretation: _____

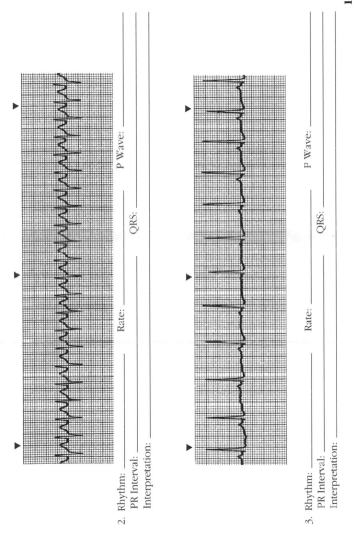

2. Rhythm: _____ Rate: _____ P Wave: _____
   PR Interval: _____ QRS: _____
   Interpretation: _____

3. Rhythm: _____ Rate: _____ P Wave: _____
   PR Interval: _____ QRS: _____
   Interpretation: _____

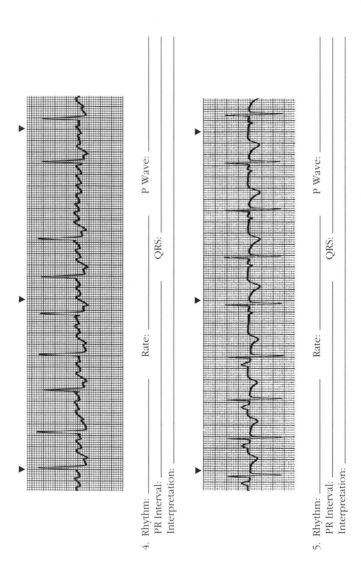

4. Rhythm: _____ Rate: _____ P Wave: _____

   PR Interval: _____ QRS: _____

   Interpretation: _____

5. Rhythm: _____ Rate: _____ P Wave: _____

   PR Interval: _____ QRS: _____

   Interpretation: _____

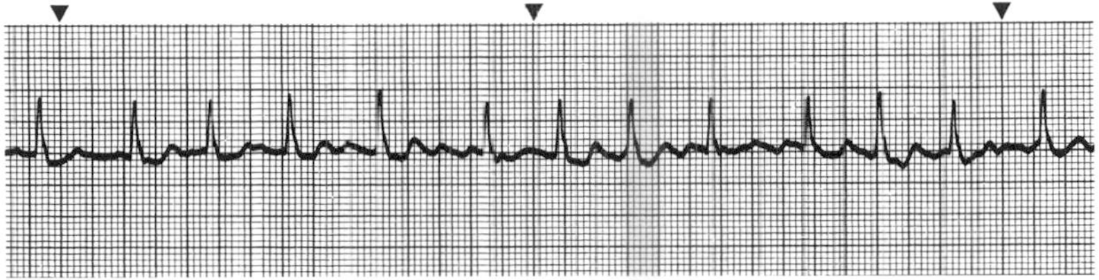

6. Rhythm: _____ Rate: _____ P Wave: _____

   PR Interval: _____ QRS: _____

   Interpretation: _____

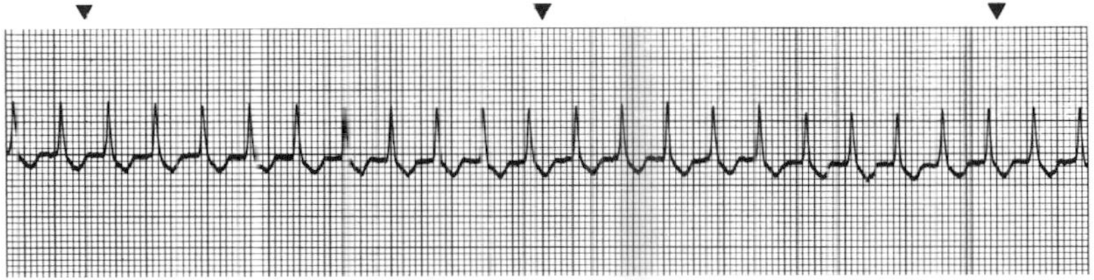

7. Rhythm: _____ Rate: _____ P Wave: _____

   PR Interval: _____ QRS: _____

   Interpretation: _____

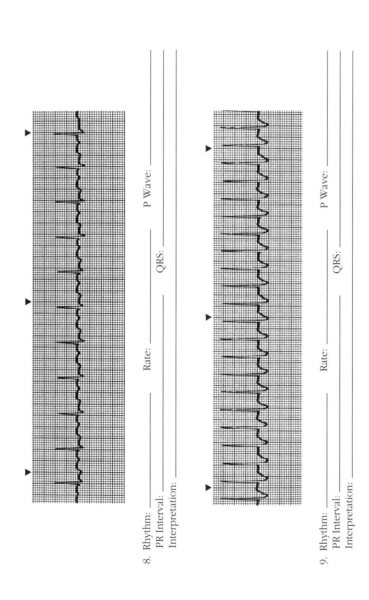

8. Rhythm: _____ Rate: _____ P Wave: _____
   PR Interval: _____ QRS: _____
   Interpretation: _____

9. Rhythm: _____ Rate: _____ P Wave: _____
   PR Interval: _____ QRS: _____
   Interpretation: _____

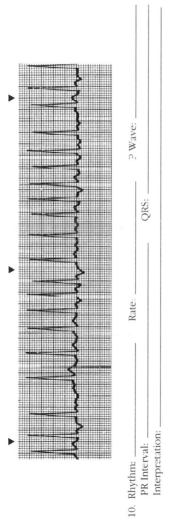

10. Rhythm: _____ Rate: _____ P Wave: _____
    PR Interval: _____ QRS: _____
    Interpretation: _____

CHAPTER EIGHT
AV JUNCTIONAL ARRHYTHMIAS AND BLOCKS

If the SA node is suppressed as a result of increased parasympathetic activity or cardiac pathology, the AV node can function as a pacemaker, firing about 60 to 75 beats/min. The pacemaker cells in the junctional tissue surrounding the AV node (junctional pacemakers) can fire between 40 and 60 beats/min. A cardiac rhythm originating from these cells, an ectopic focus, is called a *junctional rhythm*. After you complete this chapter, you should be able to identify four AV junctional rhythms: premature junctional contractions, paroxysmal junctional tachycardia, AV junctional escape beats, and junctional escape rhythms.

Although AV blocks occur anywhere from the SA node to the Purkinje fibers, the AV node is the most common site. These blocks are diagnosed by examining the P wave in relation to the QRS complex; the PR interval is a major indicator of the degree of blockage present. Three types of AV block are presented here: first-degree, second-degree, and third-degree heart block.

AV Junctional Rhythms

When AV junctional tissue takes over firing the impulse for atrial depolarization, the impulse must travel "backward" up to the atria. This is called *retrograde conduction*. This conduction produces inverted P waves in positive ECG leads, especially lead II, and upright deflections in negative leads. The ventricles are depolarized in the normal way.

The AV junctional rhythms can be premature and accelerated. The three characteristic P wave patterns depend on the priority of atrial and ventricular depolarization.

1. If the junctional impulse depolarizes the atria first, followed by ventricular depolarization, the *P wave* will *precede* the QRS complex (Fig. 8-1**A**).

2. If the junctional impulse triggers both atrial and ventricular depolarization at the same time, then the *P wave* is *hidden* in the QRS complex (Fig. 8-1**B**).

3. If the junctional impulse depolarizes the ventricles first, followed by the atria, the *P wave* will *follow* the QRS complex (Fig. 8-1**C**).

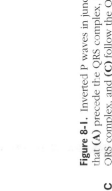

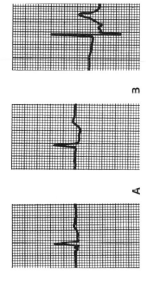

Figure 8-1. Inverted P waves in junctional arrhythmias that **(A)** precede the QRS complex, **(B)** are hidden in the QRS complex, and **(C)** follow the QRS complex.

Premature Junctional Contractions

A premature junctional contraction (PJC) occurs when an irritable junctional focus discharges an impulse before the SA node fires. Abnormal P waves can precede, follow, or occur simultaneously with the QRS complex. Ventricular contraction is usually normal. PJCs are not very common and not very dangerous. Usually they are only singular beats interrupting the heart's regular pattern. They are often followed by an incomplete or complete compensatory pause. PJCs can lead to premature atrial contractions (PACs).

Occasionally, a PJC will occur late in the cycle and be referred to as a junctional escape beat. These beats, though not requiring treatment, need to be accurately identified.

ETIOLOGY

A PJC can occur in healthy individuals with no history of heart disease.

- Cardiac disease: CAD, CHF, rheumatic heart disease, MI
- Diet: caffeine-containing beverages (coffee, soda, tea)
- Emotions: anxiety, excitement, fear, stress
- Life-style: exercise, excessive use of alcohol or tobacco

SYMPTOMS

Most individuals are asymptomatic.

- Cardiac: feelings of palpitations, fluttering, or a "skipped beat"

Primary Treatment Goals

Treatment depends on eliminating or managing the cause of the PJCs.

- Cardiac drugs: quinidine sulfate
- Modifying diet and life-style
- Reducing stress

Arrhythmia Characteristics

- Rate: usually normal, depends on the rate of the basic rhythm, can be bradycardic or tachycardic
- Rhythm: usually irregular
- P waves: pattern depends on atrial and ventricular depolarization. P waves may be abnormal, premature (precede the QRS complex), can occur after the QRS complex, or can be hidden within the QRS. P waves will be inverted in positive leads and upright in negative leads.
- PR interval: may be less than 0.12 second; pattern depends on P wave position.
- QRS complex: normal

SAMPLE ECG STRIP

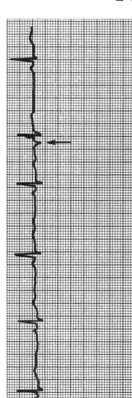

Figure 8-2. Premature junctional contractions.

Paroxysmal Junctional Tachycardia

Paroxysmal junctional tachycardia (PJT) arises from an ectopic focus that is strong enough to take over the pacemaker activity of the heart (Fig. 8-3). It is usually defined as a cluster of three or more PJCs, rapidly firing at a rate of more than 150 beats/min. Accurate diagnosis is important because premature atrial tachycardia (PAT) looks similar to PJT.

ETIOLOGY

The condition has the same causes that stimulate PJCs, especially acute cardiac disease, although PJTs can occur in persons without a cardiac history.

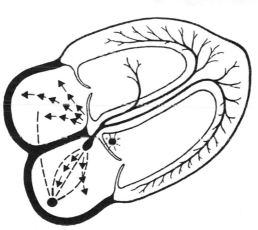

Figure 8-3. Cardiac illustration of paroxysmal junctional tachycardia.

SYMPTOMS

- Asymptomatic at rates less than 150 beats/min
- Cardiac (at rates > 150 beats/min): chest pain and pressure, palpitations
- Neurologic: dizziness, syncope

PRIMARY TREATMENT GOALS

The goal is to establish normal SA node activity.

- Cardioversion if warranted
- Medications: calcium channel blockers, CNS depressants, digoxin
- Vagal stimulation maneuvers (carotid sinus massage, Valsalva maneuver)

ARRHYTHMIA CHARACTERISTICS

- Rate: usually greater than 100 beats/min; can be as high as 250 beats/min
- Rhythm: usually regular
- Conduction: regular to slightly irregular
- P waves: inverted in positive leads and upright in negative leads; may be hidden in rates greater than 150 beats/min
- PR interval: less than 0.12 second, especially if P waves precede QRS
- QRS complex: usually normal

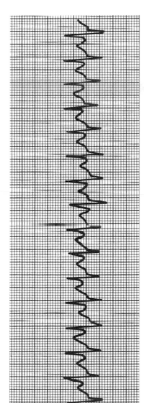

Figure 8-4. Paroxysmal junctional tachycardia.

AV Junctional Escape Beat

An AV junctional escape beat occurs when the AV junction takes over the pacemaker activity of the heart; the SA node fails to discharge an impulse or the impulse is blocked in the atrial conduction system. These beats occur late in the cardiac cycle and prevent the heart from stopping completely. The AV junctional rate is about 40 to 60 beats/min. The P waves are usually inverted in lead II and may occur before, during, or after a QRS complex.

ETIOLOGY

- Cardiac disease: rheumatic heart disease, MI
- Common sinus arrhythmias: sinus bradycardia, sinus block, and sinus arrest
- Failure of the SA node to fire or blockage of impulses by the SA node
- Medications: β blockers, calcium channel blockers, CNS depressants, digoxin, narcotics, sedatives

SYMPTOMS

Most individuals are asymptomatic.

- Feelings of palpitations, fluttering, or a "skipped beat"

PRIMARY TREATMENT GOALS

Most treatment measures are those used for sinus bradycardia; some are nonspecific.

ARRHYTHMIA CHARACTERISTICS

- Rate: normal, bradycardic, or tachycardic
- Rhythm: regular to slightly irregular
- Conduction: usually normal
- P waves: inverted in lead II, either precede, follow, or hidden in the QRS complex
- PR interval: usually less than 0.11 second, especially if PR interval precedes the QRS complex
- QRS complex: usually normal

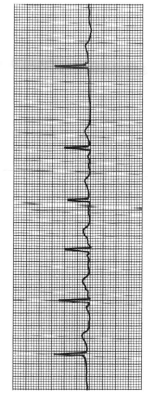

Figure 8-5. Junctional escape beat.

Junctional Escape Rhythm

A junctional escape rhythm is a cluster of four or more junctional escape beats that follow each other. The beats occur when the AV junction takes over the pacemaker role of the heart because the SA node has failed to fire or its impulse is blocked. This rhythm is seen in conditions such as sinus bradycardia and sinus arrest.

The junctional escape rhythm discharges at a rate of 40 to 60 beats/min. The rate decreases cardiac output and may lead to other cardiac conditions. As with the escape beats, P waves may precede, follow, or be hidden in the QRS complex. The P waves will be inverted in positive leads and upright in negative leads.

ETIOLOGY

The etiology is similar to that for AV junctional escape beats.

SYMPTOMS

Most individuals are asymptomatic if the rate stays greater than 50 beats/min.

- Cardiac (at rate < 50 beats/min): chest pain or pressure, dyspnea, hypotension, palpitations
- Neurologic: dizziness, syncope, unconsciousness

ARRHYTHMIA CHARACTERISTICS

- Rate: 40 to 60 beats/min
- Rhythm: regular to slightly irregular
- Conduction: normal yet delayed with a heart rate of 40 to 60 beats/min
- P waves: inverted in positive leads and upright in negative leads; P waves can occur before, during, or after QRS complex.
- PR interval: less than 0.12 second if P wave precedes QRS complex
- QRS complex: usually normal

SAMPLE ECG STRIP

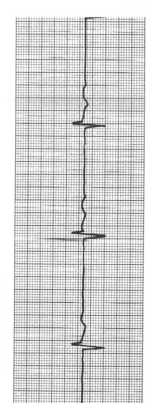

Figure 8-6. Junctional escape rhythm.

AV Blocks

First-Degree Block

A first-degree AV block is characterized by a *delay* in the conduction at the AV node for more than 0.2 second. The impulse spreads normally from the SA node. Despite the delay, every impulse makes it through to the ventricles. Even though this conduction abnormality is a delay and not a true block, the term block is still used.

AV Junctional Arrhythmias and Blocks

ETIOLOGY

- Common occurrence in normal hearts
- Beginning degenerative disease of the conduction system
- Cardiac disease: arteriosclerotic heart disease, myocarditis, organic heart disease, after MI tissue injury to AV node or surrounding tissue
- Medications: β blockers, calcium antagonists, digitalis toxicity

SYMPTOMS

Symptoms are usually not evident.

PRIMARY TREATMENT GOALS

Treatment is usually not necessary unless the block is caused by medication that can be modified or withheld.

ARRHYTHMIA CHARACTERISTICS

- Rate: 60 to 100 beats/min, depending on rhythm
- Rhythm: usually regular
- Conduction: delayed with prolonged PR intervals greater than 0.2 second
- P waves: normal, one P wave for every QRS complex
- PR interval: greater than 0.2 second
- QRS complex: usually normal, follows every P wave

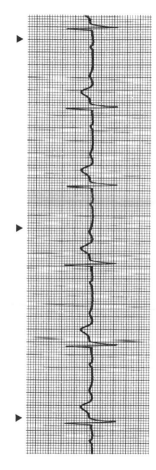

Figure 8-7. Normal sinus rhythm with first-degree heart block.

Second-Degree Block

Second-degree AV block is characterized by an interruption in impulse conduction, not just a delay. Impulses from the atrial areas never reach the ventricles. This is seen on the ECG by the presence of P waves not followed by QRS complexes. The two forms of second-degree AV block are distinguished by the PR interval. The two types are: Mobitz type I (Wenckebach) block and Mobitz type II.

135

MOBITZ TYPE I (WENCKEBACH) AV BLOCK

This block is the least serious and most common of the second-degree blocks. It usually never progresses to third-degree blockage. The characteristic pattern to this block is easily recognized on an ECG strip.

This block is within the AV node. Each successive impulse produces a longer and longer delay in the AV node until the third or fourth impulse cannot make it through to the ventricles. The ECG strip shows the PR interval getting *progressively longer* until finally a P wave occurs without a QRS complex. This is referred to as a "dropped beat." This pattern continues to repeat itself. This ratio of P waves to the QRS complexes can be abbreviated as 5:4, 4:3, or 3:2.

ETIOLOGY

- Always associated with some type of heart disease, especially ischemic injury to AV node and surrounding tissue secondary to an injury
- Same conditions that cause first-degree AV block

SYMPTOMS

Symptoms depend on the rhythm and degree of blockage and usually subside in 3 to 4 days.
- Cardiac: an irregular heart rate, an occasional "skipped" beat, chest pain and pressure, dizziness, hypotension

Primary Treatment Goals

Treatment is not necessary unless the block is caused by medication that can be modified or withheld.

- Medications: IV atropine or dopamine to increase heart rate
- Permanent pacemaker insertion may be required.

Arrhythmia Characteristics

- Rate
  - Atrial: 60 to 100 beats/min
  - Ventricular: slower than the atrial rate; depends on ratio of P waves to QRS complexes (5:4, 4:3, 3:2)
- Rhythm: usually slow; atrial rhythm regular, ventricular rhythm: irregular
- Conduction: some impulses do not conduct through to the ventricles
- P waves: more P waves than QRS complexes
- PR interval: progressively prolongs until dropped beat occurs
- QRS complex: usually normal except for "dropped beats"

SAMPLE ECG STRIP

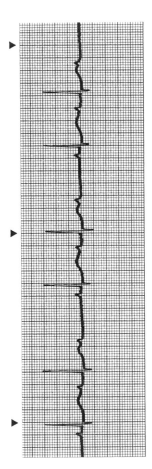

Figure 8-8. Second-degree AV block, type I.

MOBITZ TYPE II AV BLOCK

This block is more serious than the Wenckebach AV block because the blockage is below the AV node in the bundle of His or the bundle branch area. The impulse can progress rapidly to a more serious blockage, specifically third-degree AV block or asystole. The ECG strip shows the PR intervals to be of a *constant length* prior to the dropped QRS complex. The ratio of P waves to QRS complexes varies constantly (4:3, to 3:2, to 2:1).

ETIOLOGY

- Same conditions that cause first-degree AV block
- Usually always associated with cardiac disease, especially an MI that causes ischemia to tissues around the bundle of His or the bundle branch area

SYMPTOMS

The patient is asymptomatic if AV block is not significant.

- Cardiac (related to diminished cardiac output): chest pain and pressure, dyspnea, hypotension, lethargy
- Neurologic: dizziness, syncope, unconsciousness

PRIMARY TREATMENT GOALS

- Aggressive management is necessary to prevent progression to third-degree blockage: IV atropine increases atrial contractions, thus subsequently increasing ventricular contractions and increasing the speed of impulses.
- Medications: CNS stimulants. IV dopamine if severe hypotension is present
- Temporary transvenous pacemaker will be necessary when the arrhythmia is identified.

ARRHYTHMIA CHARACTERISTICS

- Rate and conduction: same as Mobitz type I

- Rhythm: atrial rhythm regular, ventricular rhythm may or may not be regular depending on whether or not there is a consistent block
- P waves: more P waves than QRS complexes
- PR interval: can be longer than normal
- QRS complex: normal if defect is in the bundle of His; greater than 0.12 second if bundle branch block exists

SAMPLE ECG STRIP

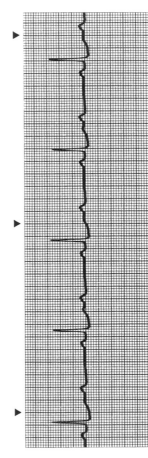

Figure 8-9. Second-degree AV block, Mobitz type II.

Third-Degree Block

Third-degree AV block is also called *complete heart block* because no atrial impulses get through to the ventricles. The blockage is below the AV node in the bundle of His or the bundle branch area. When this happens, the atria and ventricles continue to beat at their intrinsic rate, each being driven by an independent pacemaker. The atria and ventricles continue to beat at their intrinsic rate, each being driven by an independent pacemaker. The atria beat at 60 to 100 beats/min. The ventricles beat at 20 to 60 beats/min. If the pacemaker site is at the AV junction (junctional pacemaker) then the ventricular rate follows the normal ventricular conduction pathways and ranges from 40 to 60 beats/min. If the pacemaker site originates in the ventricles, then there is no normal conduction pathway and the ventricular rate is about 20 to 40 beats/min.

ETIOLOGY

- Cardiac disease: CAD, CHF, degenerative heart disease, MI
- Medications: β blockers, calcium channel blockers, digitalis toxicity

SYMPTOMS

Symptoms are directly related to the ventricular rate and the amount of activity and exercise tolerance.

- Cardiac: chest pressure and pain, dyspnea, hypotension, lethargy
- Neurologic: syncope, unconsciousness

PRIMARY TREATMENT GOALS

It is rare that a patient can tolerate this arrhythmia, but it is possible if the ventricular rate is adequate.

- Medications: IV atropine sulfate, isoproterenol, or dopamine
- Temporary or permanent transvenous pacemaker insertion

ARRHYTHMIA CHARACTERISTICS

- Rate
  - Atrial: 60 to 100 beats/min
  - Ventricular: 20 to 60 beats/min depending on ventricular pacemaker site
- Rhythm: atrial and ventricular regular but at separate rates
- Conduction: no atrial impulses are conducted to the ventricles, ventricular beats are ectopic with varying to nonexistent patterns.
- P waves: hidden within QRS complexes and T waves
- PR interval: variable
- QRS complex: if originating in the AV junction then a regular pattern occurs that is not associated with P waves; if the QRS is of ventricular origin then the complexes are greater than 0.12 second.

SAMPLE ECG STRIP

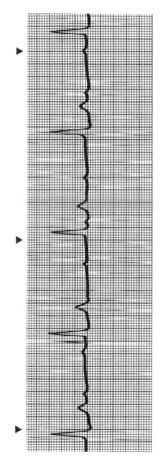

Figure 8-10. Third-degree AV block.

Unit Summary

This unit ends the three chapters specific to arrhythmias of sinus and atrial origin. You should now know how to identify basic arrhythmia patterns and know when to report significant information to a health care professional. The practice rhythm strips should have reinforced or clarified information as needed. You now have the foundation to move on to recognizing ventricular arrhythmias.

Practice Rhythm Strip Analysis

Examine each of the following 16 sample AV junctional rhythms and blocks. Identify each arrhythmia and describe significant characteristics. Write your answers on the lines provided.

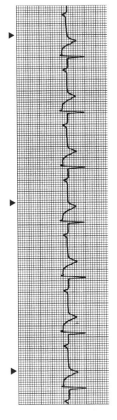

1. Rhythm: _____ Rate: _____ P Wave: _____

   PR Interval: _____ QRS: _____

   Interpretation: _____

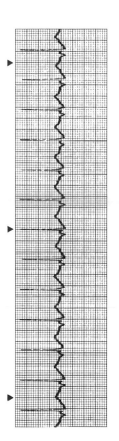

2. Rhythm: _____ Rate: _____ P Wave: _____
   PR Interval: _____ QRS: _____
   Interpretation: _____

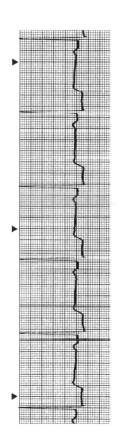

3. Rhythm: _____ Rate: _____ P Wave: _____
   PR Interval: _____ QRS: _____
   Interpretation: _____

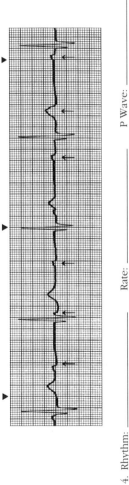

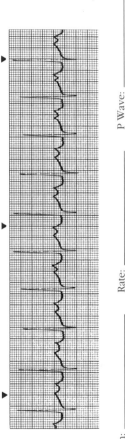

4. Rhythm: _____ Rate: _____ P Wave: _____
   PR Interval: _____ QRS: _____
   Interpretation: _____

5. Rhythm: _____ Rate: _____ P Wave: _____
   PR Interval: _____ QRS: _____
   Interpretation: _____

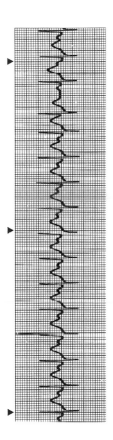

6. Rhythm: _____ Rate: _____ P Wave: _____

   PR Interval: _____ QRS: _____

   Interpretation: _____

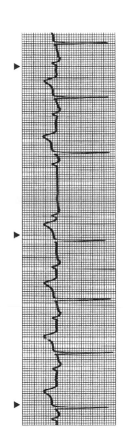

7. Rhythm: _____ Rate: _____ P Wave: _____

   PR Interval: _____ QRS: _____

   Interpretation: _____

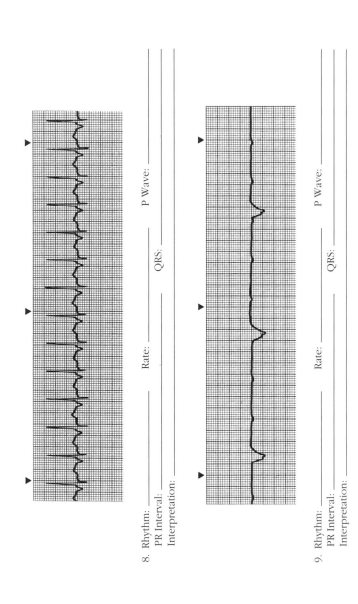

8. Rhythm: _____   Rate: _____   P Wave: _____
   PR Interval: _____   QRS: _____
   Interpretation: _____

9. Rhythm: _____   Rate: _____   P Wave: _____
   PR Interval: _____   QRS: _____
   Interpretation: _____

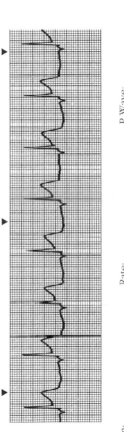

▶ ▶ ▶

10. Rhythm: _____ Rate: _____ P Wave: _____
    PR Interval: _____ QRS: _____
    Interpretation: _____

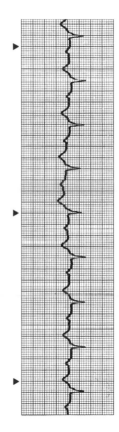

▶ ▶ ▶

11. Rhythm: _____ Rate: _____ P Wave: _____
    PR Interval: _____ QRS: _____
    Interpretation: _____

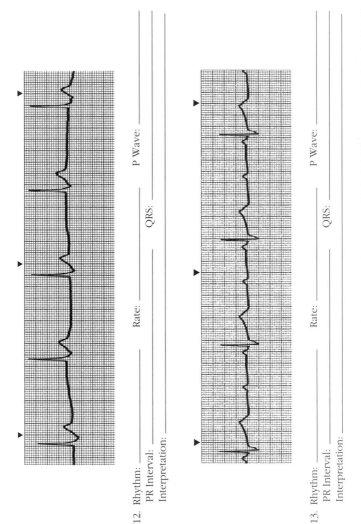

12. Rhythm: _____ Rate: _____ P Wave: _____

PR Interval: _____ QRS: _____

Interpretation: _____

13. Rhythm: _____ Rate: _____ P Wave: _____

PR Interval: _____ QRS: _____

Interpretation: _____

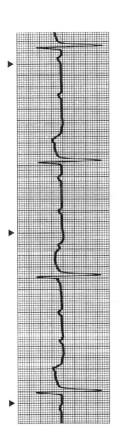

14. Rhythm: _____ Rate: _____ P Wave _____

    PR Interval: _____ QRS: _____

    Interpretation: _____

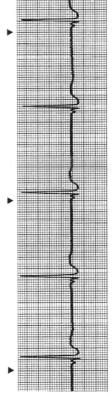

15. Rhythm: _____ Rate: _____ P Wave: _____

    PR Interval: _____ QRS: _____

    Interpretation: _____

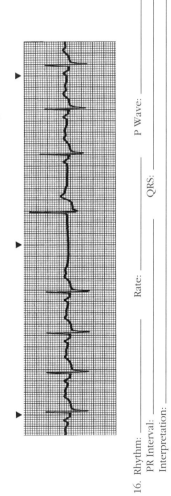

16. Rhythm: _____   Rate: _____   P Wave: _____
    PR Interval: _____   QRS: _____
    Interpretation: _____

Unit IV

Chapter 9
Ventricular Arrhythmias

Chapter 10
Cardiac Disease:
Angina Pectoris and MI

Arrhythmias and Cardiac Disease Affecting the Ventricles

The previous three units have prepared you for the next level of identifying several potentially life-threatening ventricular arrhythmias that can result in decreased cardiac output and subsequent cardiac failure. The *most serious* ventricular arrhythmias are those associated with left ventricular damage.

Ventricular arrhythmias are potentially lethal because they are the result of changes in the heart's tissue caused by cardiac disease. Cardiac disease, the *major cause* of morbidity and mortality in the United States today, primarily affects the coronary arteries and the heart's musculature, the myocardium.

The dangerous accumulation of lipid (fat) materials in the coronary arteries lead to narrowed vessel lumens and obstructed blood flow. Diminished blood flow through the coronary arteries results in insufficient oxygen flow to the myocardium, a condition known as *ischemia*. Ischemia can progress to cellular tissue damage.

Cellular death of myocardial tissue (infarction) causes conduction abnormalities and the ineffective mechanical pumping of the heart's chambers. The most common and most critical areas of infarction occur in the left ventricle. Ventricular infarctions can quickly lead to death, in 3 to 5 minutes, or to a lifetime of chronic illness.

In this unit, six ventricular arrhythmias are presented: premature ventricular contractions, ventricular tachycardia, ventricular flutter, ventricular fibrillation, asystole, and ventricular escape beats. Practice rhythm strips are provided to improve the rapid recognition and interpretation of these potentially lethal arrhythmias. Analysis of sample rhythm patterns follows the same format used in Unit III.

CHAPTER NINE
VENTRICULAR ARRHYTHMIAS

Ventricular arrhythmias are the *most serious* of all arrhythmias. Rapid firing and incomplete ventricular contractions result in the insufficient filling of the ventricles with blood. This causes compromised blood flow to the pulmonary artery and the aorta. Frequently, depolarizations are so slow that cardiac output is insufficient to meet the body's circulatory and metabolic needs. Ventricular pacemaker sites are also dangerous because they may take over the heart's electrical conduction.

Long-term and continued decreased cardiac output can eventually lead to cardiac failure. When you complete this chapter, you should be able to identify these five common ventricular arrhythmias: premature ventricular contractions, ventricular tachycardia, ventricular flutter, ventricular fibrillation, and asystole. Additionally, ventricular escape beats are discussed, although this arrhythmia is not as common as the others.

Premature Ventricular Contractions

Premature ventricular contractions (PVCs) are the result of an irritable focus in one of the ventricles that discharges an impulse before a regularly scheduled impulse is received from the SA node (Fig. 9-1). The rhythm of the heart is interrupted. The QRS complex is wider than 0.10 second and may be

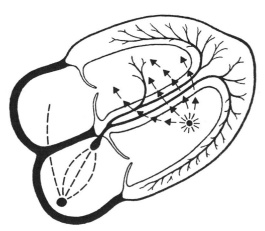

Figure 9-1. Cardiac illustration of premature ventricular contractions.

bizarre in appearance. The P wave may or may not be present because the SA node is not affected by the PVCs. The T wave is inversely proportional (equal yet opposite direction) to the QRS deflection, that is, if the T wave is inverted, then the QRS is upright. PVCs occur along with other rhythms, such as bradycardia and tachycardia. A PVC may be singular or occur every two, three, or four beats. Three or more PVCs constitute ventricular tachycardia.

The PVC, the *most common* of all ventricular contractions, produces little or no cardiac output because of inadequate ventricular filling. Approximately 80% of all post-MI patients will experience PVCs because sensitive areas of cardiac tissue are damaged from myocardial ischemia or injury. This is always of grave concern for this population because PVCs can signal the onset of ventricular tachycardia or ventricular fibrillation, which can be life-threatening. Occasionally a ventricular escape beat will occur with characteristics similar to the PVC; however, these escape beats require no treatment.

ETIOLOGY

- Cardiac disease: CAD, CHF, MI
- Diet: caffeine-containing beverages (coffee, soda, tea)
- Electrolyte disturbances: hypermetabolic states, hypokalemia
- Emotions: anxiety, excitement, fear, stress
- Life-style: exercise, excessive use of alcohol or nicotine
- May occur in a healthy individual with no prior history of heart disease
- Medications: CNS stimulants (aminophylline, epinephrine), and OTC medications that contain stimulants (Sudafed)

SYMPTOMS

In general, most individuals state that they have the sensation of palpitations or "fluttering" in their chest. The most common complaint is the feeling of "skipped beats."

PRIMARY TREATMENT GOALS

- Treatment depends on eliminating or managing the cause of PVCs. An occasional PVC in a healthy individual will not require treatment. For the MI patient, PVCs are significant if they occur:
  - In clusters of six or more per minute
  - In pairs or groups of three
  - In every second beat
  - From a multifocal origin
  - In the vulnerable phase of electrical impulse conduction
- Medications: aggressive IV management with bretylium, lidocaine, and procainamide may be necessary for the post-MI patient or prescribed for long-term use. Lidocaine is the major drug therapy for PVCs.

ARRHYTHMIA CHARACTERISTICS

- Rate: 60 to 100 beats/min, determined by rhythm pattern, either regular or irregular
- Rhythm: regular except when PVCs occur
- Conduction: can occur backward toward the atria

- P waves: if present, may occur before or after the ectopic QRS; may be absent if the impulse originates in the ventricles
- PR interval: determined by the basic rhythm
- QRS complex: may be normal, premature, wide (> 0.10 second), or bizarre depending on the number of ventricular foci; usually not associated with a P wave

SAMPLE ECG STRIPS

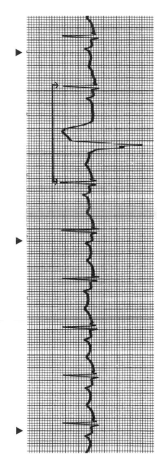

Figure 9-2. Normal sinus rhythm with one premature ventricular contraction.

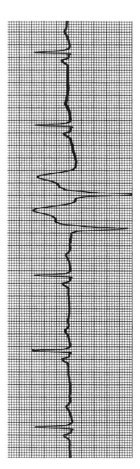

Figure 9-3. Paired premature ventricular contractions.

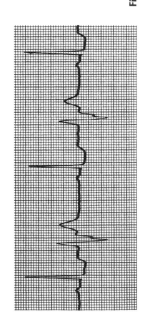

Figure 9-4. Bigeminal premature ventricular contractions.

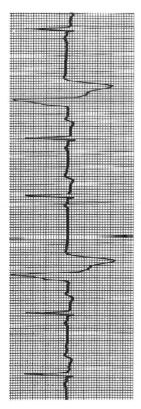

Figure 9-5. Trigeminal premature ventricular contractions.

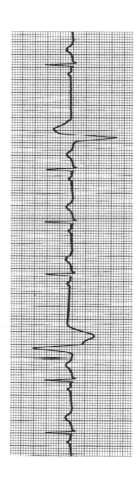

Figure 9-6. Multifocal premature ventricular contractions.

Ventricular Tachycardia

Ventricular tachycardia (also called V-tach), caused by a single, rapid, and irritable ventricular focus, is considered the *most dangerous* of all ventricular arrhythmias. This arrhythmia is similar to a grouping of multiple PVCs that significantly decrease cardiac output and can result in death. The degree of seriousness depends on the duration of the arrhythmia. Prolonged ventricular tachycardia can progress to ventricular fibrillation.

ETIOLOGY

- Cardiac disease: CAD, CHF, MI
- Causes similar to those of PVCs
- Electrolyte disturbances: acidosis, hypokalemia
- Extrinsic causes: cardiac catheterization procedures, central venous pressure lines, electrical shock, pacemaker insertion, pulmonary artery catheters, and unexpected and sharp blows to the chest
- Medications: cardiac drugs (digoxin, quinidine), CNS stimulants, thyroid medications

SYMPTOMS

- Cardiac: absence of pulse, chest pressure and pain, dyspnea, hypotension, sense of "fluttering" in the chest, and tachycardia
- Neurologic: loss of consciousness and pupil dilation

Primary Treatment Goals

Treatment depends greatly on the severity of the arrhythmia and the patient's degree of tolerance.

- CPR
- Electrical cardioversion is the treatment of choice for rapid termination of beats when patients are not responsive to drug therapy.
- Insertion of a temporary pacemaker
- Implantable defibrillator for long-term prevention
- Management or elimination of the underlying cause
- Medications: aggressive IV therapy with drugs (bretylium, procainamide, and lidocaine)

Arrhythmia Characteristics

- Rate: 150 to 250 beats/min
- Rhythm: regular or slightly irregular
- Conduction: originates in the ventricles so the impulse can occur backward toward the atria
- P waves: usually hidden in the QRS complex
- PR interval: not measurable
- QRS complex: similar to PVCs, wide and bizarre with T wave in opposite direction

SAMPLE ECG STRIP

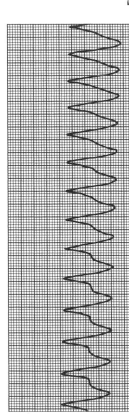

Figure 9-7. Ventricular tachycardia.

Ventricular Flutter

This arrhythmia is so similar to ventricular tachycardia that little time will be spent on it here. Basically, ventricular flutter arises from an irritable focus in the ventricles that acts as a ventricular pacemaker. This irritability is more pronounced than that found in ventricular tachycardia yet less severe than that found in ventricular fibrillation.

ETIOLOGY AND SYMPTOMS

These are the same as those for ventricular tachycardia.

Primary Treatment Goals

Treatments are the same as those for ventricular tachycardia except treatment needs to be rapid because ventricular fibrillation may quickly occur. Electrical cardioversion is usually the initial treatment.

Arrhythmia Characteristics

- Rate: greater than 250 beats/min
- Rhythm: regular to slightly irregular
- Conduction: no organized conduction because of rapidly firing foci
- P waves: not usually present
- PR interval: not measurable
- QRS complex: rounded, stretched "slinky" appearance

SAMPLE ECG STRIP

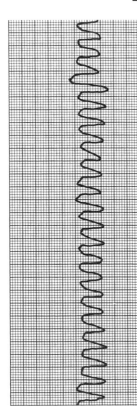

Figure 9-8. Ventricular flutter.

Ventricular Fibrillation

Ventricular fibrillation is a lethal arrhythmia because effective circulation virtually stops. It is the *most common* cause of death in patients who have CAD. The ventricles cannot contract because of the rapidity of the electrical impulse. The ventricles "quiver" such that no effective cardiac output can occur. The quivering is usually stimulated by PVCs or ventricular tachycardia (Fig. 9-9).

ETIOLOGY

Ventricular fibrillation is caused by the same factors that cause ventricular tachycardia.

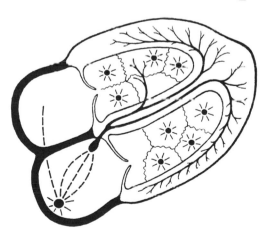

Figure 9-9. Cardiac illustration of ventricular fibrillation.

SYMPTOMS

- Cardiac: absence of pulse, blood pressure, and respirations; cardiac and respiratory arrest, cold and clammy skin, cyanosis
- Neurologic: immediate unconsciousness with convulsions secondary to decreased or absent cerebral blood flow

PRIMARY TREATMENT GOALS

- Cardiac drugs: antiarrhythmic agents after fibrillation has stopped
- Electrical defibrillation
- Immediate initiation of CPR within 1 to 2 minutes

ARRHYTHMIA CHARACTERISTICS

- Rate: too rapid to count
- Rhythm: irregular and uncoordinated
- Conduction: no organized conduction
- P waves: not visible
- PR interval: not measurable
- QRS complex: a quivering, nondistinct pattern

SAMPLE ECG STRIP

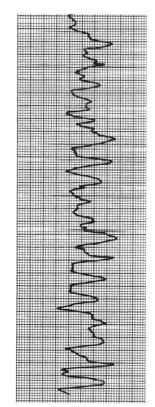

Figure 9-10. Ventricular fibrillation.

Asystole

Asystole is the absence of a heart rate with no cardiac output. Ventricular contraction ends and circulation stops. The patient becomes unconscious and death occurs in a few minutes.

ETIOLOGY

Asystole is preceded by other lethal ventricular arrhythmias and is indicative of death.

SYMPTOMS

- Cardiac: absence of pulse, blood pressure, and respirations' cyanosis
- Neurologic: fixed and dilated pupils

PRIMARY TREATMENT GOALS

Determine if treatment is desirable. Monitored, terminally ill patients may request no resuscitative measures.

- Distinguish from ventricular fibrillation
- If a straight line suddenly appears on an ECG tracing then CPR is quickly initiated (make sure an artifact, such as a dislocated lead, has not caused the straight line).
- CPR will be followed with intubation and IV medications, such as atropine, epinephrine, and sodium bicarbonate.

ARRHYTHMIA CHARACTERISTICS

- Rate: no ventricular rate; an inherent apical slow beat may occur.
- Rhythm: no electrical activity
- Conduction: absent
- P wave: may be present but not likely
- PR interval: not measurable
- QRS complex: not present

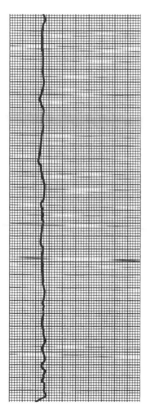

Figure 9-11. Asystole.

Ventricular Escape Beats

Ventricular escape beats appear when regular atrial depolarization fails to occur due to a blockage at the SA node. There is a resultant pause in the cardiac cycle. Escape beats occur after a pause. When the AV junction fails to function as a pacemaker, then the ventricles initiate an impulse, usually from the Purkinje fibers. These ventricular beats prevent asystole.

ETIOLOGY

- Any condition that interferes with normal impulse generation by the SA node
- Medical conditions that result in bradycardia

SYMPTOMS

- Cardiac symptoms related to decreased output: cyanosis, dyspnea, hypotension, sensation of "skipped beats"

PRIMARY TREATMENT GOALS

There is no specific treatment. The primary goal is to increase circulation. Note: *never* give IV lidocaine to patients with ventricular escape beats because the lidocaine may completely stop ventricular contractions.

ARRHYTHMIA CHARACTERISTICS

- Rate: usually less than 60 beats/min; may be normal
- Rhythm: regular or irregular
- Conduction: abnormal; escape beats occur after regular impulse is not produced.
- P waves: present or absent; P wave does not precede escape beat.
- PR interval: depends on rhythm
- QRS complex: underlying rhythm may be normal or QRS wider than 0.12 second. Escape beat is greater than 0.12 second.

SAMPLE ECG STRIP

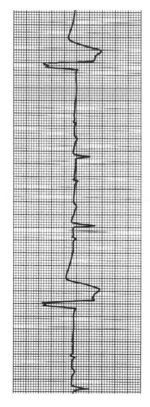

Figure 9-12. Ventricular escape beats.

Practice Rhythm Strip Analysis

Examine each of the following 12 sample arrhythmias of ventricular origin. Identify each arrhythmia and describe significant characteristics. Write your answers on the lines provided.

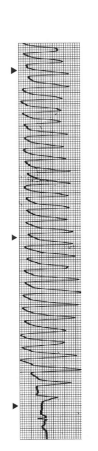

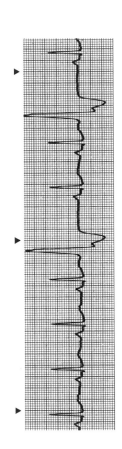

1. Rhythm: _____ Rate: _____ P Wave: _____
   PR Interval: _____ QRS: _____
   Interpretation: _____

2. Rhythm: _____ Rate: _____ P Wave: _____
   PR Interval: _____ QRS: _____
   Interpretation: _____

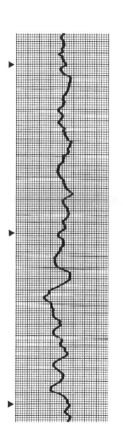

3. Rhythm: _____ Rate: _____ P Wave _____
   PR Interval: _____ QRS: _____
   Interpretation: _____

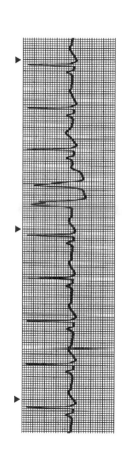

4. Rhythm: _____ Rate: _____ P Wave: _____
   PR Interval: _____ QRS: _____
   Interpretation: _____

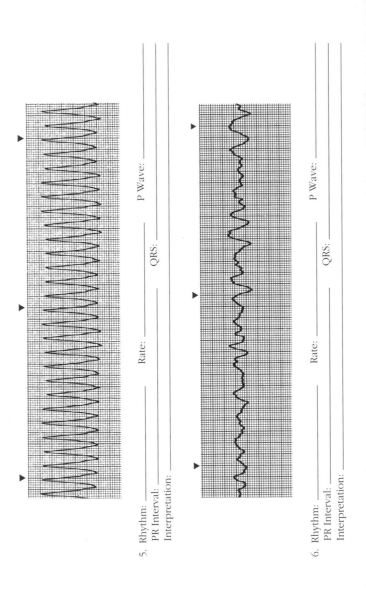

5. Rhythm: _____   Rate: _____   P Wave: _____
   PR Interval: _____   QRS: _____
   Interpretation: _____

6. Rhythm: _____   Rate: _____   P Wave: _____
   PR Interval: _____   QRS: _____
   Interpretation: _____

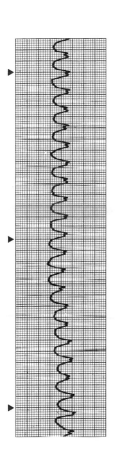

▶

▶

▶

7. Rhythm: _____ Rate: _____ P Wave: _____
   PR Interval: _____ QRS: _____
   Interpretation: _____

8. Rhythm: _____ Rate: _____ P Wave: _____
   PR Interval: _____ QRS: _____
   Interpretation: _____

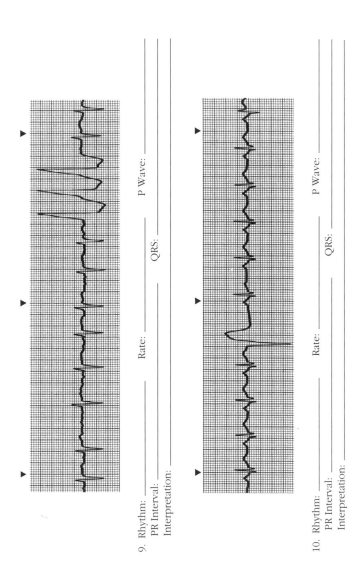

9. Rhythm: _____ Rate: _____ P Wave: _____
   PR Interval: _____ QRS: _____
   Interpretation: _____

10. Rhythm: _____ Rate: _____ P Wave: _____
    PR Interval: _____ QRS: _____
    Interpretation: _____

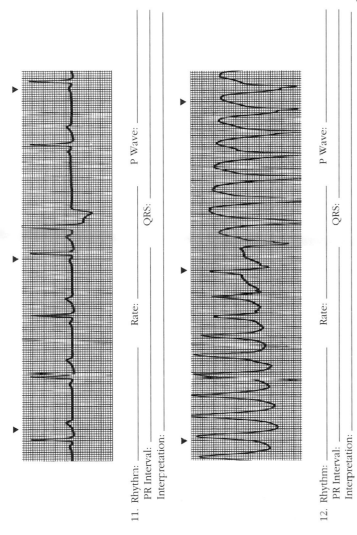

11. Rhythm: _____ Rate: _____ P Wave: _____
    PR Interval: _____ QRS: _____
    Interpretation: _____

12. Rhythm: _____ Rate: _____ P Wave: _____
    PR Interval: _____ QRS: _____
    Interpretation: _____

179

CHAPTER TEN
CARDIAC DISEASE: ANGINA PECTORIS AND MI

With cardiac disease, irreversible damage occurs when the myocardial tissue is deprived of an adequate supply of oxygen. This tissue damage is identified by the area of the left ventricle where the cellular necrosis and death has occurred. The most common infarcted areas of the left ventricle are identified as the anterior, lateral, inferior, and posterior walls. In this chapter, you will learn how to identify infarcted tissue on an ECG. You will also learn what leads to review for specific areas of infarct damage.

Angina Pectoris

Coronary atherosclerosis, the *most common* heart disease in the United States, leads to coronary artery narrowing, which causes decreased blood flow and oxygen to the myocardium. Diminished oxygenation of the left ventricular myocardial tissue is called *ischemia.* Ischemia can be noted on an ECG strip when the T wave is inverted and the ST segment is depressed (Fig. 10-1).

T Wave Inverted

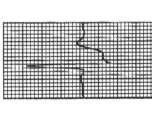

ST Depression

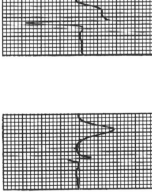

Figure 10-1. Ischemic changes on an ECG tracing.

REMEMBER

When reviewing an ECG strip, the T wave is normally inverted in leads III, aVR, and V_1.

181

An MI or "heart attack" occurs when coronary artery circulation is shut off to a portion of the heart's tissue. Although an MI occurs in any area of the heart, most MIs occur in the left ventricle. A thrombus or coronary artery spasm usually causes the sudden cessation of circulation.

The two major coronary arteries (right coronary and left coronary) supply oxygenated blood to specific areas of the heart. An occlusion or spasm in any one of these arteries causes damage to a specific area of the heart. MIs are referred to by the section of the left ventricle that is damaged, either the anterior, lateral, inferior, or posterior wall (Chart 10-1 and Fig. 10-2).

Posterior MIs are recorded on an ECG strip in leads directly over the region of tissue damage. When an area of myocardial tissue dies, it can no longer generate electrical activity. When the infarcted area is in the left ventricle, the electrical activity from the right ventricle becomes dominant and three characteristic ECG wave patterns appear. These patterns are usually progressive and any one characteristic may occur without the others.

Use Chart 10-2 and Figure 10-3 to review lead placement over specific regions of the heart. If necessary, refer back to Chapter 2 for a review of lead placements.

ECG Changes With an MI

T WAVE INVERSION

T wave inversion is an indicator of *ischemia*; it cannot be used solely to diagnose an MI. Occasionally inverted T waves are preceded by tall and narrow (peaked or hyperactive) T waves that eventu-

Chart 10-1. Coronary Artery Supply to Specific Areas of Myocardium That Are Affected by Infarctions

Coronary Artery	Coronary Artery Blood Supply to Ventricular Area	Infarcted Region Dependent on Coronary Artery Blood Supply
Left Coronary Artery		
Anterior descending	Along the anterior section of the left ventricle	Anterior
Circumflex	Upper lateral wall of left ventricle and left atrium	Lateral
Right Coronary Artery		
	Right ventricle	
Posterior descending branch	Inferior section of left ventricle	Inferior
	Posterior section of left ventricle	Posterior

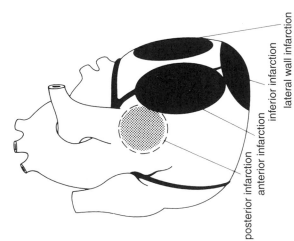

Figure 10-2. Anatomic sites of myocardial infarction.

Chart 10-2. ECG Leads Directly Over Regions Where a Myocardial Infarction Is Localized

Region of Heart Where Infarction Is Localized	Precordial and Limb Leads Directly Over Infarcted Region
Anterior: anterior surface of left ventricle	V_1 through V_6
Lateral: the left lateral wall of the heart	I, aVL, V_5 and V_6
Inferior: the area of the diaphragmatic surface of the heart	II, III, and aVF
Posterior: posterior surface of the heart	No specific leads Reciprocal changes can be seen in V_1, V_2, and V_3

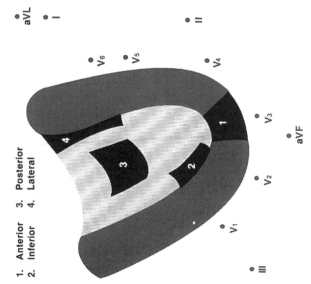

Figure 10-3. Locations of myocardial infarction relative to ECG lead placements.

1. Anterior   3. Posterior
2. Inferior   4. Lateral

ally invert. Their origin and significance is not completely understood. Since ischemia is reversible, T waves will convert to normal with the return of adequate oxygenation, which can occur in 2 hours or within several months (Fig. 10-4). Sometimes T waves remain inverted for months or years.

ST SEGMENT ELEVATION

ST segment elevation is an indicator of *injury*, usually cellular damage, when found in leads placed over the infarcted area. Initially an elevated ST segment may merge with the T wave, a good indicator that MI has occurred These elevations usually return to baseline 3 to 4 days after the beginning of symptoms (Fig. 10-5).

SIGNIFICANT Q WAVES

Significant Q waves are waves that are more than 0.04 second in duration, exceed the height of the R wave by 30% (> 2 mm), and are found in leads placed over an infarcted area (Fig. 10-6). Significant Q waves usually occur within hours of an injury and may last forever because necrosis represents irreversible tissue injury.

REMEMBER

 Deep Q waves can be normally seen in lead aVR and are not diagnostic of an MI. Non-Q wave infarctions do occur. They are associated with an ECG strip that shows T wave inversion and ST segment depression.

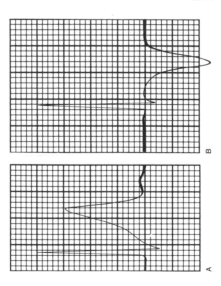

Figure 10-4. T wave response (**A**) during and (**B**) 2 hours after a myocardial infarction.

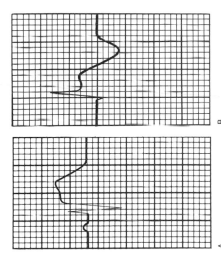

A   B

Figure 10-5. Examples of ST segment elevation during an acute myocardial infarction: (**A**) without T wave inversion; (**B**) with T wave inversion.

RECIPROCAL CHANGES

The three manifestations of ECG changes just reviewed (T wave inversion, ST segment elevation, and the presence of significant Q waves) occur when leads are placed over an infarcted area. ECG changes are also seen in leads placed over areas opposite the infarcted region (Chart 10-3). Three *reciprocal changes* are: tall T waves, depressed ST segments, and R waves that exhibit increased height.

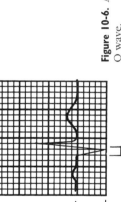

Figure 10-6. A significant Q wave.

Regional Infarcts

You have now learned how to recognize specific ECG changes indicative of an MI. You have also learned which coronary artery or branch is responsible for specific regional infarcts. Following are examples of ECG changes in all relevant leads for each of the four primary regional infarcts: anterior, lateral, inferior, and posterior.

ANTERIOR WALL INFARCTION

Significant Q waves may not always be present. In some patients, the diagnostic criteria may be an abnormal pattern of R wave progression (Fig. 10-7, p. 192).

LATERAL WALL INFARCTION

See Figure 10-8, p. 193, for significant Q waves in four leads.

Chart 10-3. ECG Leads Opposite Region Where Myocardial Infarction Is Localized

Region of Heart Where Infarction Is Localized	Precordial and Limb Leads Directly Over Infarcted Region	Precordial and Limb Leads Opposite the Infarcted Area
Anterior: anterior surface of left ventricle	V_1 through V_6	II, III, and aVF are reciprocal to V_5 and V_6
Extensive Anterior	V_1 through V_5	No reciprocal leads
Septal	V_1 and V_2	
Anterior	V_3 and V_4	
Lateral: the left lateral wall of the heart	I, aVL, V_5 and V_6	II, III, and aVF
Inferior: the area of the diaphragmatic surface of the heart	II, III, and aVF	I, aVL, V_5 and V_6
Posterior: posterior surface of the heart	No specific leads. Reciprocal changes can be seen in V_1, V_2, and V_3	V_1, V_2, and V_3

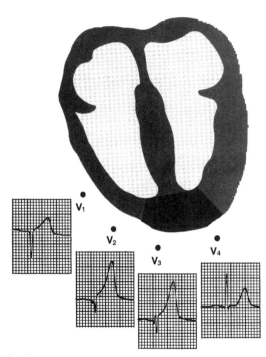

Criterion

Q waves in V₁ – V₄

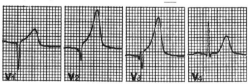

Figure 10-7. Significant Q waves identifiable in leads V₁ through V₄.

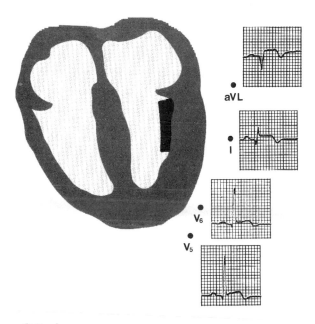

Criterion

Q waves in I, aVL, V$_5$, and V$_6$

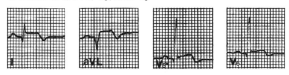

Figure 10-8. Significant Q waves are identifiable in leads I, aVL, V$_5$, and V$_6$.

INFERIOR WALL INFARCTION

With this type of infarction, significant Q waves may persist forever or disappear in 6 to 9 months. Smaller Q waves may represent an old MI or may be normal in some hearts (Fig. 10-9).

POSTERIOR WALL INFARCTION

Since no leads lie over this area of the heart, reciprocal changes need to be identified in the anterior leads. Diagnostic changes include elevated R waves and depressed ST segments in leads V_1 and V_2 (Fig. 10-10).

Unit Summary

You have now completed one of the most challenging units in this book—challenging in that the content is complex and the responsibility for the recognition and interpretation of these arrhythmias is enormous. Please use these units periodically for review.

You should now have the basic understanding of distinguishing common ventricular arrhythmias, arrhythmias of a sinus and atrial origin, and arrhythmias arising from AV junctions. The next two units cover the remaining miscellaneous arrhythmias frequently encountered in clinical practice.

Practice Rhythm Strip Analysis

Examine and identify each of the four sample infarctions (pps. 197–200.). Write your answers on the lines provided.

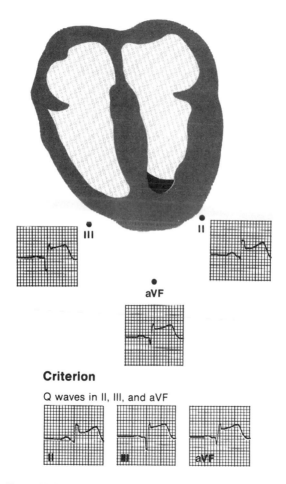

Criterion

Q waves in II, III, and aVF

Figure 10-9. Significant Q waves in leads II, III, and aVF.

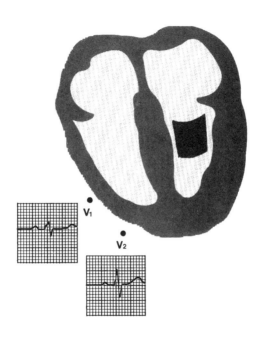

Criterion

Tall R waves in V_1 and V_2 often accompanied by tall T waves

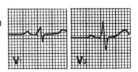

Figure 10-10. Tall or elevated R waves in V_1 and V_2. Elevated T waves are present sometimes.

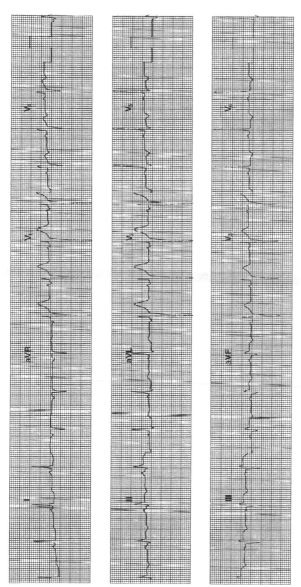

1. Infarction: _____

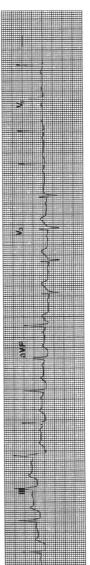

2. Infarction: _____

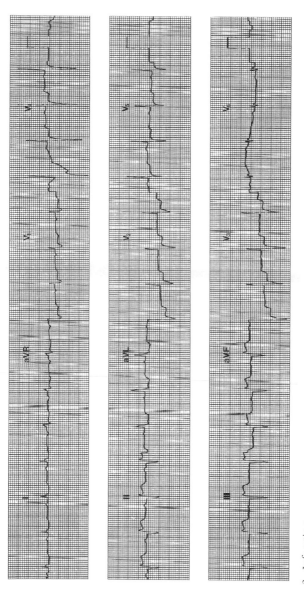

3. Infarction: _____

4. Infarction: _____

Chapter 11
Bundle Branch Blocks

Chapter 12
Arrhythmias Caused by Electrolytes and Medications

Miscellaneous Arrhythmias

To develop competency in the recognition of arrhythmias, it is important to have a comprehensive understanding of all arrhythmias, including those not classified by either their atrial or ventricular origins. In this unit, you will learn how to distinguish arrhythmias caused by the conduction abnormalities associated with bundle branch blocks as well as miscellaneous arrhythmias caused by electrolytes and medications.

Bundle branch blocks are divided into right bundle branch blocks, left bundle branch blocks, hemiblocks, and alternating and intermittent blocks. Electrolyte abnormalities are limited to the common ECG patterns seen with abnormalities in potassium and calcium, two electrolytes that can have significant and lethal effects on the heart.

The effects of three medications (digitalis, procainamide, and quinidine) on ECG rhythms are presented to help you learn how to distinguish a therapeutic pattern from a dangerous arrhythmia. As with the previous units, sample rhythm strips are used to illustrate ECG patterns and analysis exercises are provided.

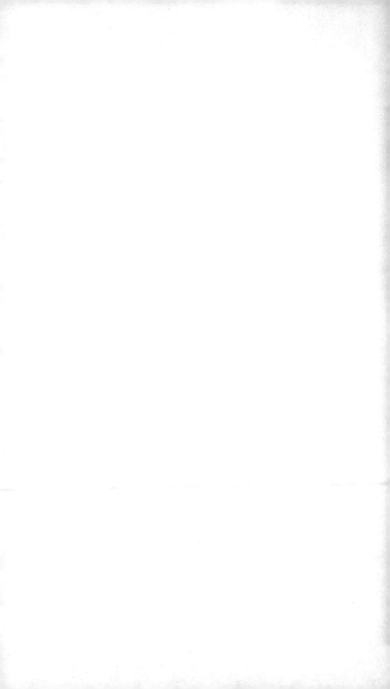

CHAPTER ELEVEN
BUNDLE BRANCH BLOCKS

Bundle branch blocks are easy to interpret on the ECG once you understand the underlying conduction abnormality. By now you know that the normal sequence of ventricular depolarization represented by a QRS complex is narrow and less than 0.10 second. When blockage exists in the bundle branches, the conduction system compensates by depolarizing the unblocked side first. The impulse then travels across the interventricular septum to next depolarize the ventricle with the blocked bundle branch. The result of this altered conduction pathway is separate ventricular depolarizations that produce altered and prolonged QRS complexes (usually > 0.12 second).

These bundle branch blocks can be temporary or permanent. Two types are presented here: right bundle branch block (RBBB) and left bundle branch block (LBBB). Hemiblocks and alternating or intermittent blocks are briefly explained.

Right Bundle Branch Block

In RBBB, the electrical impulse is blocked through this bundle. Therefore the impulse initially travels down the unblocked left bundle branch and depolarizes the left ventricle first (Fig. 11-1). As this is happening, the impulse then travels across the interventricular septum and then depolarizes the right ventricle. This delay in right ventricular depolarization causes a widened QRS complex (> 0.12 second). The QRS complex takes on a distinct pattern of a second R wave (R'). A jagged-type appearance is reflected on the ECG, frequently referred to as "rabbit ears," which is very diagnostic in precordial leads V_1 and V_2. Additionally, you may find T wave inversion and depression of the ST segment.

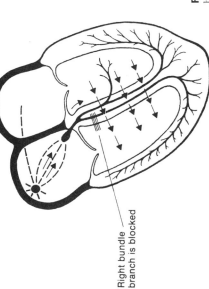

Right bundle branch is blocked

Figure 11-1. Cardiac illustration of right bundle branch block.

ETIOLOGY

- Cardiac disease: arteriosclerotic heart disease, CAD, CHF, chronic obstructive pulmonary disease, congenital anomalies for children, MI; can be found in normal hearts

SYMPTOMS

Symptoms are usually not evident because the heart rate and rhythm are not affected.

PRIMARY TREATMENT GOALS

Treatment is usually not necessary unless the block is caused by medications that can be modified or withhe.d.

ARRHYTHMIA CHARACTERISTICS

- Rate usually within normal range; depends on rhythm
- Rhythm: regular or irregular; depends on rate
- Conduction: usually normal
- P waves: may be present or absent depending on rhythm
- PR interval: usually normal
- QRS complex: less than 0.12 second an additional R' wave as depolarization moves toward V_1 and an S wave as depolarization moves away from lead I (Fig. 11-2).

SAMPLE ECG STRIP

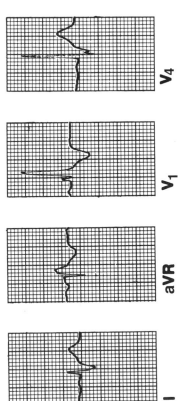

I   aVR V_1 V_4

Figure 11-2. A right bundle branch pattern.

Left Bundle Branch Block

In LBBB the reverse of RBBB occurs. The electrical impulse travels down the RBBB initially and depolarizes the right ventricle first (Fig. 11-3). The impulse then travels across the interventricular septum and depolarizes the left ventricle. This delay in left ventricular depolarization causes a widened QRS complex (> 0.12 second). The QRS complex takes on a distinct pattern of a very elongated R

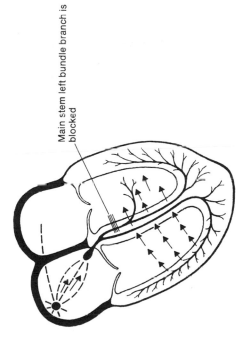

Figure 11-3. Cardiac illustration of left bundle branch block.

Main stem left bundle branch is blocked

207

wave that is inverted in the leads over the left ventricle (I, aVL, V_5, and V_6). Additionally, T wave inversion and ST segment depression can be seen. It is essential that this block be accurately interpreted because it obscures the ECG changes reflected with MI.

ETIOLOGY

- Rarely occurs in normal hearts
- Cardiac disease (CAD, CHF, MI) and conduction abnormalities

SYMPTOMS

Symptoms are usually not evident because the heart rate and rhythm are not affected.

PRIMARY TREATMENT GOALS

Treatment is usually not necessary unless the block is caused by medications that can be modified or withheld.

ARRHYTHMIA CHARACTERISTICS

- Rate: usually within normal range; depends on rhythm
- Rhythm: regular or irregular, depending on rate
- Conduction: usually normal
- P waves: may be present or absent depending on rhythm
- PR interval: usually normal
- QRS complex: more than 0.12 second; widened and bizarre, predominately negative in V_1 (Fig. 11-4)

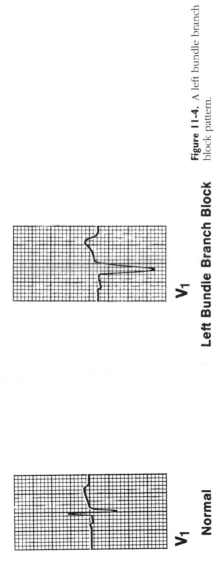

V₁

Normal

V₁

Left Bundle Branch Block

Figure 11-4. A left bundle branch block pattern.

Hemiblock

A hemiblock refers to an electrical conduction blockage that occurs in one of the three fascicles (little bundles of nerve fibers) of the left bundle branch (Fig. 11-5). It is presented here for your infor-

209

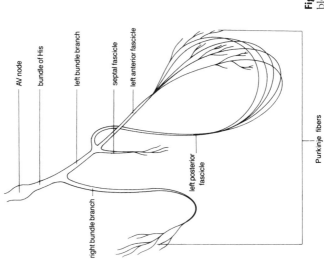

Figure 11-5. Fascicles that can evidence a blockage.

mation. However, its identification and interpretation on the ECG strip requires a more detailed analysis than is the purpose of this book.

Alternating or Intermittent Blocks

Alternating blocks exist when RBBBs and LBBBs alternate in groups of beats. This pattern can be seen when wide QRS complexes alternate positive and negative presentations (Fig. 11-6). Intermittent

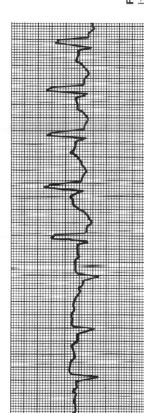

Figure 11-6. An alternating bundle branch block.

blocks exist when RBBBs or LBBBs (or both) are intermittently placed among normal QRS complexes (Fig. 11-7). The etiology, symptomatology, and treatment goals are similar to the bundle branch blocks.

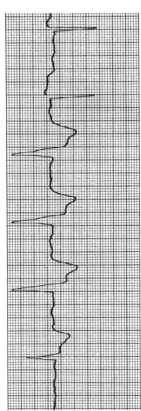

Figure 11-7. An intermittent bundle branch block.

Practice Rhythm Strip Analysis

Examine each of the following eight sample bundle branch block arrhythmias. Identify each arrhythmia and describe significant characteristics. Write your answers on the lines provided.

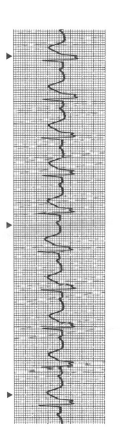

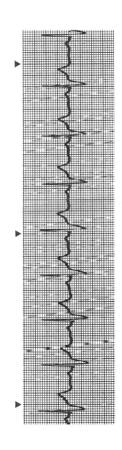

1. Rhythm: _____ Rate: _____ P Wave: _____
   PR Interval: _____ QRS: _____
   Interpretation: _____

2. Rhythm: _____ Rate: _____ P Wave: _____
   PR Interval: _____ QRS: _____
   Interpretation: _____

213

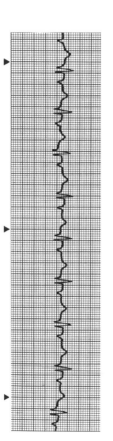

3. Rhythm: _____ Rate: _____ P Wave: _____
   PR Interval: _____ QRS: _____
   Interpretation: _____

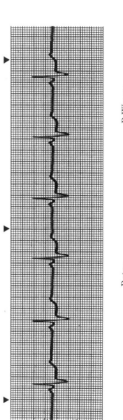

4. Rhythm: _____ Rate: _____ P Wave: _____
   PR Interval: _____ QRS: _____
   Interpretation: _____

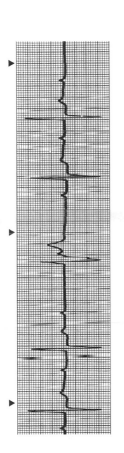

5. Rhythm: _____   Rate: _____   P Wave: _____

   PR Interval: _____   QRS: _____

   Interpretation: _____

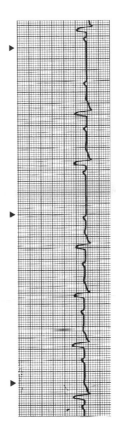

6. Rhythm _____   Rate: _____   P Wave: _____

   PR Interval: _____   QRS: _____

   Interpretation: _____

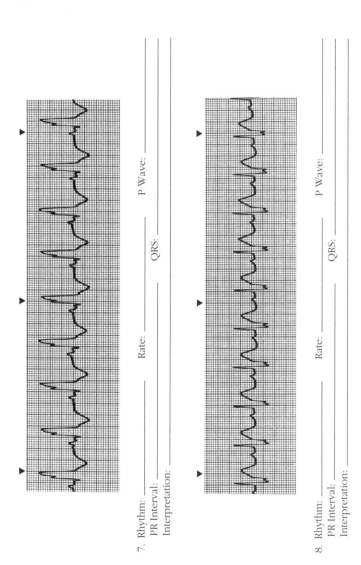

7. Rhythm: _____ Rate: _____ P Wave: _____
   PR Interval: _____ QRS: _____
   Interpretation: _____

8. Rhythm: _____ Rate: _____ P Wave: _____
   PR Interval: _____ QRS: _____
   Interpretation: _____

CHAPTER TWELVE
ARRHYTHMIAS CAUSED BY ELECTROLYTES AND MEDICATIONS

Electrolyte disturbances and certain antiarrhythmic medications alter the normal pattern of the ECG. Some changes are expected, some are indicative of significant changes in the patient's medical condition, and some are indicators of arrhythmias that, if left unchecked, can become life-threatening. The role of the health care provider is to analyze the rhythm strip, recognize and interpret changes, and report significant information.

The variety of noncardiac or cardiac disorders and medications affecting ECG rhythms is too extensive to be presented here, for example, electrolyte disturbances, medical conditions (hypothermia), cardiac disorders (myocarditis, pericarditis), pulmonary embolism, and CNS disease (cerebral anoxia and hemorrhage). For the sake of brevity and relevance, only two major electrolytes and three primary antiarrhythmic drugs are reviewed.

Electrolyte Abnormalities

Potassium (normal serum level is 3.5–5.5 mEq/L) and calcium (normal serum level is 8.5–10.5 mg/dL) imbalances can cause significant ECG changes, primarily with the ST segment and the T wave. Most of these changes are the result of action potentials that are somewhat altered.

Hypokalemia

Hypokalemia can be defined as a serum potassium level less than normal. The ECG pattern is characterized by a prominent U wave (the *most definite* indicator of hypokalemia), a flattened T wave that often merges with the U wave, and ST segment depression (Fig. 12-1).

Hyperkalemia

Hyperkalemia can be defined as a serum potassium level higher than normal. The ECG pattern reflects progressive changes consistent with increases in serum potassium. Tall, peaked T waves that resemble tents, especially in the precordial leads, are initially indicative of hyperkalemia. Diffuse changes in the T waves distinguish this pattern from the pattern seen with an MI.

As potassium levels rise, the T wave elongates along with the QRS complex; the P and R waves become flat in appearance. Eventually the deflections form a characteristic "sine wave" pattern (Fig. 12-2). Hyperkalemic manifestations on an ECG tracing warrant immediate medical attention.

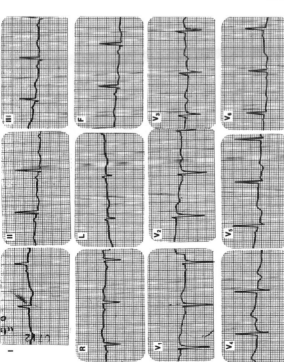

Figure 12-1. An ECG pattern indicative of hypokalemia.

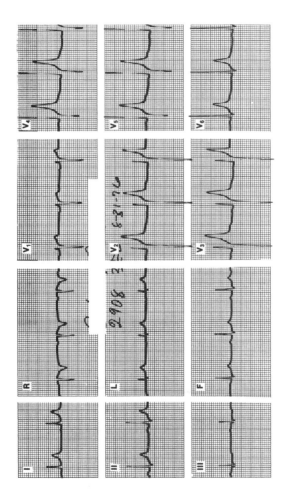

Figure 12-2. An ECG pattern indicative of hyperkalemia.

Hypocalcemia and Hypercalcemia

Alterations in serum calcium levels are evidenced on the ECG by changes in the QT interval; hypocalcemia prolongs the QT interval and hypercalcemia shortens the QT interval. These changes are influenced by alterations in the ST segment; the T wave is rarely affected (Fig. 12-3).

Medication Effects

A variety of medications can cause significant changes in ECG patterns, all in some way affecting action potentials. Antiarrhythmic drugs, administered for the therapeutic medical management of cardiac arrhythmias, alter ECG rhythm patterns. However, toxic drug levels and side effects, which are potentially lethal, should be immediately interpreted and reported so intervention can occur. The

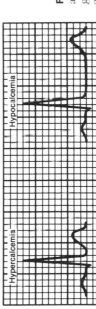

Figure 12-3. An ECG pattern indicative of hypercalcemia and hypocalcemia. The magnitude of the QT change generally is proportional to the severity of the calcium abnormality.

three most significant drugs that can produce toxic drug levels are digitalis, quinidine, and procainamide.

Digitalis

Digitalis, an antiarrhythmic and cardiac glycoside, therapeutically increases the force of myocardial contraction, decreasing conduction throughout the SA and AV nodes. This action causes expected ECG pattern changes: ST segment depression and T wave inversion in leads with positive QRS complexes. The ST segment presents a "scooped" appearance (Fig. 12-4). Nontherapeutic levels can lead to arrhythmias such as first-, second-, and third-degree AV block and atrial and ventricular tachyarrhythmias (paroxysmal atrial tachycardia and premature ventricular contractions are common).

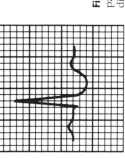

Figure 12-4. An ECG pattern influenced by digitalis.

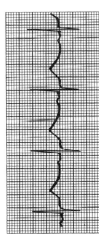

Figure 12-5. An ECG pattern reflecting a prolonged QT interval subsequent to the effects of quinidine.

Quinidine and Procainamide

Quinidine and procainamide, both potent antiarrhythmic drugs, slow conduction velocity and decrease myocardial excitability. For patients taking these drugs, the ECG shows prolonged QT intervals, inverted T waves, and depressed ST segments. These drugs can cause serious side effects when dosage levels become toxic. A prolonged QT interval (> 25%) is cause for alarm (Fig. 12-5).

Unit Summary

This unit concludes the presentation of miscellaneous arrhythmias. Common ECG changes seen with conduction abnormalities found with bundle branch blocks were reviewed. Arrhythmias resulting from abnormal electrolyte levels for potassium and calcium and adverse reactions to three commonly prescribed antiarrhythmic medications were presented. You are encouraged to refer to additional reference materials for a more detailed analysis of miscellaneous conduction abnormalities not within the scope of this book.

Unit VI

Pacemaker Therapy and Continuous Cardiac Monitoring

This final unit addresses pacemaker therapy and cardiac monitoring. The differences between internal, external, temporary, and permanent pacemakers are explained. Key terms used to clarify ECG patterns caused by a pacemaker are defined and the system of coding is outlined in a chart. Sample ECG rhythm strips that illustrate pacemaker influence are presented.

The final chapter presents the equipment and lead placement positions necessary for continuous cardiac monitoring. Various types of artifacts are explained and sample rhythm strips are provided to illustrate the influence of artifacts on ECG patterns.

Chapter 13
Pacemaker Therapy and ECG Patterns

Chapter 14
Continuous Cardiac Monitoring

CHAPTER THIRTEEN
PACEMAKER THERAPY AND ECG PATTERNS

Certain cardiac conditions, either chronic or of an emergency nature, result in the malfunctioning of an individual's electrical conduction system. Either cardiac impulses fail to discharge (sinus arrest), discharge too slowly (bradycardia), discharge too rapidly (tachyarrhythmias), fail to conduct (AV block), or are refractory to medications. When the heart's internal pacemaker functions fail, an electrical impulse can be delivered by an artificial pacemaker, an electronic device that provides repetitive electrical stimuli to the heart to cause ventricular contraction.

Types of Pacemakers

Pacemakers can be external or internal. This chapter focuses on internal pacing systems. However, before beginning, it is important to understand that, in emergency situations, where transvenous access is not possible, external pacing is an important adjunct to therapy. With external pacing, electrode pads are strategically placed on the anterior and posterior chest walls such that an electrical charge can stimulate the myocardium (Fig. 13-1).

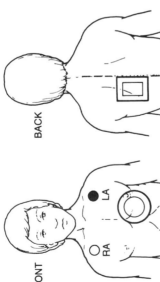

FRONT

RA ○   ● LA

BACK

Figure 13-1. External pacemaker electrode placement.

Internal pacemakers are either *temporary* or *permanent*. Basically, a pacemaker has two parts: an electronic pulse generator that contains batteries and electrical wires, and the pacemaker electrodes or leads that carry electrical stimuli to the heart. Pulse generators are powered by batteries (mercury-zinc, lithium, or plutonium) that last from 3 to 20 years or longer. Pacemakers function on demand or at a fixed rate.

Demand pacemakers stimulate the heart "on demand," when the ventricles do not normally repolarize and the heart rate drops below a certain rate. *Fixed-rate pacemakers* stimulate ventricular contractions at a predetermined rate that is independent of the patient's rhythm. Fixed-rate pacemakers are rarely used today.

Temporary Pacemaker

Temporary transvenous pacing is done as an emergency procedure and is used for days, weeks, or months until a permanent pacemaker can be inserted. Temporary pacemakers are usually necessary for patients with significant bradycardia, heart block, or cardiac arrest. Temporary pacing can be transvenous or transthoracic.

With a transvenous pacemaker, the pacing electrode is inserted, threaded under fluoroscopy through a venous route (ie, antecubital, brachial, subclavian), and positioned in the apex of the right ventricle (Fig. 13-2). The temporary transvenous demand pacemaker is the *most common* approach used today for acute cardiac disorders especially after an MI.

Permanent Pacemaker

Permanent pacing is used for chronic conduction and rhythm disorders that cannot be managed by other means. The pacing electrode is transvenously inserted into the right ventricle (endocardial placement) or transthoracically sutured to the myocardium (epicardial placement) (Fig. 13-3). A ventricular placement is preferred. Atrial placement or atrial and ventricular placement are used if SA node stimulation is also necessary (Fig. 13-4).

The pulse generator is implanted subcutaneously underneath the skin just below the right or left clavicle; occasionally the generator is implanted in the abdominal wall. The permanent demand pacemaker is the most common type used today. It generates an electrical impulse only when the patient's intrinsic rate falls below a set threshold.

(text continues on page 233)

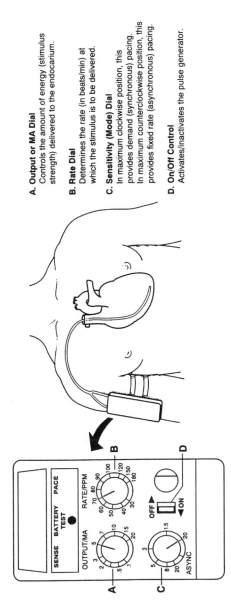

A. Output or MA Dial
Controls the amount of energy (stimulus strength) delivered to the endocarium.

B. Rate Dial
Determines the rate (in beats/min) at which the stimulus is to be delivered.

C. Sensitivity (Mode) Dial
In maximum clockwise position, this provides demand (synchronous) pacing. In maximum counterclockwise position, this provides fixed rate (asynchronous) pacing.

D. On/Off Control
Activates/inactivates the pulse generator.

Figure 13-2. A temporary pacemaker.

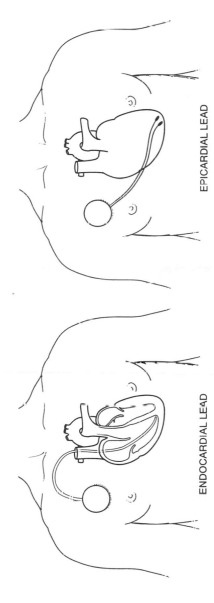

ENDOCARDIAL LEAD   EPICARDIAL LEAD

Figure 13-3. A permanent pacemaker depicting endocardial and epicardial lead placement.

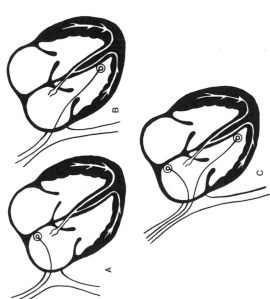

Figure 13-4. Sites of pacemaker placement.

Pacemaker Terminology and Coding

Certain key terms are used when analyzing and reporting about ECG patterns for patients with a pacemaker. It is important to understand this pacemaker language.

Key Terms

Pacemaker spike is represented by a dark line, appearing as an upward or downward deflection, just before the QRS complex in ventricular pacing and before the P wave in atrial pacing. It is an electrical artifact produced by the pacemaker.

Sensing is the ability of the electrical circuitry to distinguish the heart's intrinsic impulse generation.

Ventricular capture refers to the heart's ability to "capture" or respond to the pacing stimulus with ventricular depolarization. This will be evidenced by a *spike* in the ECG pattern, followed by a wide QRS complex.

Threshold is the amount of electrical energy needed to respond to depolarization.

A *native beat*, or intrinsic beat, is described as the beat produced by the patient's own cardiac conduction system.

A *fusion beat* is seen on the ECG when the patient's intrinsic beat occurs at the same time that the pacemaker fires (Fig. 13-5).

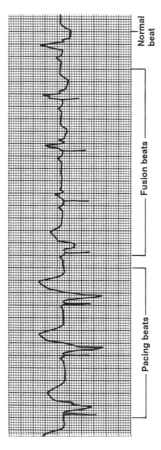

Figure 13-5. Pacemaker fusion beats.

Coding System

The International Society Commission for Heart Disease (ICHD) has identified a universal coding system to be used when describing the function of pacemakers. Each letter refers to a specific function (Chart 13-1). The first letter of the code describes the heart chamber location of the pacing electrode. The second letter describes which chamber the pacemaker generator is sensing. The final letter explains the response resulting from the pacemaker's activity. Of five possible responses, only two are common: a triggered response dependent on the heart's intrinsic rate and an inhibitory response that is controlled by the patient's heart.

Chart 13-1. TERMINOLOGY SUPPORTING ICHD CODE

Pacing Electrode Location	Chamber Being Sensed	Pacemaker Response
A—Atrium V—Ventricle D—Dual O—None	A—Atrium V—Ventricle D—Dual O—None	I—Inhibits T—Triggers D—Inhibits or Triggers O—Predetermined R—Rapid Response

ECG Patterns

In the presence of a permanent, ventricular, demand pacemaker, a small spike will appear on an ECG pattern indicating the firing of the pacemaker. This spike will appear before a wide and bizarre QRS complex. The P wave may or may not be present (Fig. 13-6). An atrial demand pacemaker will produce a spike that occurs before the P wave; the QRS complex should be normal (Fig. 13-7). Spikes

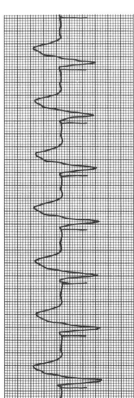

Figure 13-6. A pacing spike before a wide QRS complex.

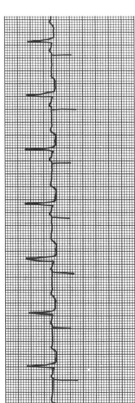

Figure 13-7. A pacing spike before a P wave.

produced by both atrial and ventricular pacemakers will be visible before each P wave and before each QRS complex (Fig. 13-8).

Pacemaker Malfunction Patterns

Three easily recognized ECG patterns reflect pacemaker malfunction: noncapture pacing or loss of capture, undersensing or non-sensing, and total pacemaker failure.

NONCAPTURE OR LOSS OF CAPTURE

Noncapture or loss of capture pacing patterns are seen when the pacemaker discharge does not produce a ventricular response. A pacemaker spike is not followed by a QRS complex (Fig. 13-9). This

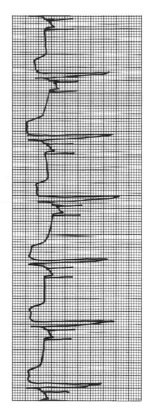

Figure 13-8. Dual pacemaker spikes produced by atrial and ventricular catheters.

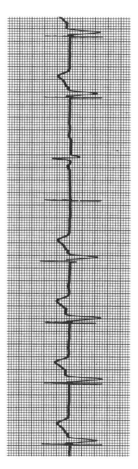

Figure 13-9. Loss of capture pacing pattern.

malfunction may be the result of an electrical threshold setting below therapeutic range or loose connections between the myocardium and the electrode tips. Treatment begins with accurate identification of the cause.

UNDERSENSING OR NON-SENSING PATTERN

An undersensing or non-sensing pattern is seen when the pacemaker does not sense the individual's intrinsic heart rate. A spiked deflection appears too early and the QRS complexes may not occur (Fig. 13-10). This malfunction may be the result of an electrical threshold setting below therapeutic range,

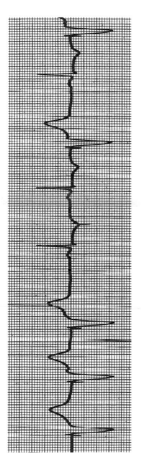

Figure 13-10. A non-sensing pacing pattern.

loose electrode connections, inaccurate catheter placement, and a malfunctioning generator. Treatment begins with accurate identification of the cause.

TOTAL PACEMAKER FAILURE

Total pacemaker failure occurs when the pacemaker stops sending impulses. An ECG pattern reflects no pacemaker spikes and no QRS complexes. This failure may be temporary or permanent and should be treated as an emergency if total failure is present.

Practice Rhythm Strip Analysis

Examine each of the following eight ECG patterns representative of normal or abnormal pacemaker functioning. Identify the automatic interval rate and describe various beats or malfunctions. Write your answers on the lines provided.

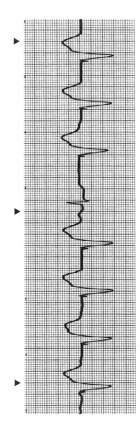
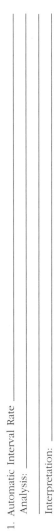

1. Automatic Interval Rate _____

   Analysis: _____

   Interpretation: _____

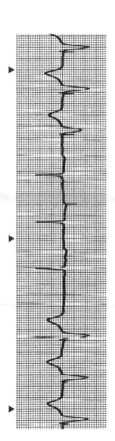

2. Automatic Interval Rate _____
   Analysis: _____

   Interpretation: _____

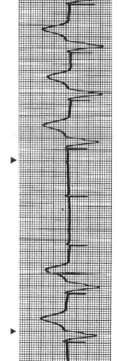

3. Automatic Interval Rate _____
   Analysis: _____

   Interpretation: _____

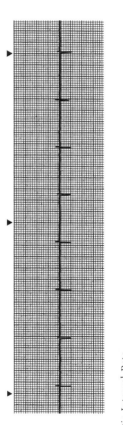

4. Automatic Interval Rate _____

    Analysis: _____

    Interpretation: _____

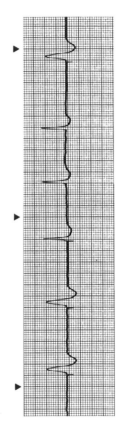

5. Automatic Interval Rate _____

    Analysis: _____

    Interpretation: _____

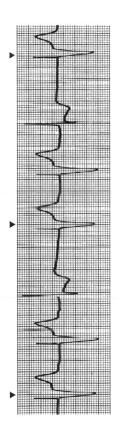

6. Automatic Interval Rate ———
   Analysis: ————————————————

   Interpretation: ————————————————

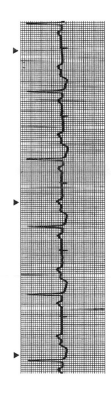

7. Automatic Interval Rate ———
   Analysis: ————————————————

   Interpretation: ————————————————

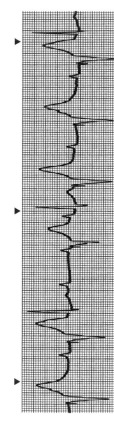

8. Automatic Interval Rate _____

   Analysis: _____

   _____

   Interpretation: _____

CHAPTER FOURTEEN
CONTINUOUS CARDIAC MONITORING

The emergence of health care finance reform and the uncontrolled growth of managed care since 1993 has significantly changed the acuity level of patients admitted to hospitals and long-term care facilities. Today, in contrast to the early 1960s, when cardiac monitors were only in critical care units, continuous cardiac monitoring is an assessment tool that is being used on many patient care floors. Physicians and licensed nursing personnel are responsible for identifying and interpreting arrhythmias. Other health care providers (patient care technicians, nursing assistants, medical assistants, registered nurses, respiratory therapists) are also responsible for monitoring continuous cardiac rhythms and reporting the appearance of arrhythmias. This chapter provides a brief overview of cardiac monitoring equipment and trouble-shooting techniques. Arrhythmia interpretation was covered in previous chapters, which you should review as necessary.

Equipment

A basic cardiac monitor (Fig. 14-1) consists of a compact unit that provides a visual display (oscilloscope) of the patient's heartbeat, which can be printed on graph paper to facilitate interpretation of

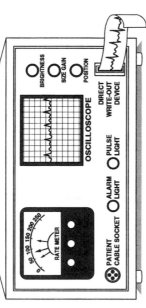

Figure 14-1. A basic cardiac monitor.

rate and rhythm. All monitors have alarm settings and light controls and are attached by electrodes to specific leads

Setting Up the Monitor

The correct placement of the cardiac monitoring leads is essential for accurate recording. Although many different systems are available, all use color codes for distinguishing between the positive and negative leads and the ground lead. Figures 14-2 and 14-3 illustrate lead placement and electrode attachment for telemetry and bedside monitoring. If you need review for understanding the basic concepts of vectors, the direction and magnitude of the heart's electrical current, the rationale for lead

(text continues on page 252)

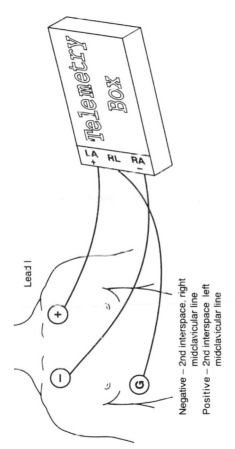

Lead I

Negative – 2nd interspace, right
midclavicular line
Positive – 2nd interspace left
midclavicular line

Figure 14-2. Electrode and lead placement for telemetry monitoring.

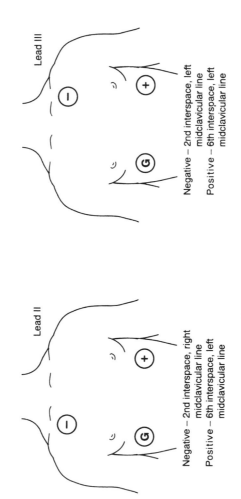

Figure 14-2. *(continued).*

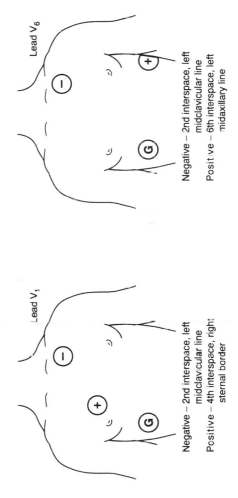

Lead V₆

Negative – 2nd interspace, left midclavicular line
Positive – 6th interspace, left midaxillary line

Lead V₁

Negative – 2nd interspace, left midclavicular line
Positive – 4th interspace, right sternal border

Figure 14-2. (continued).

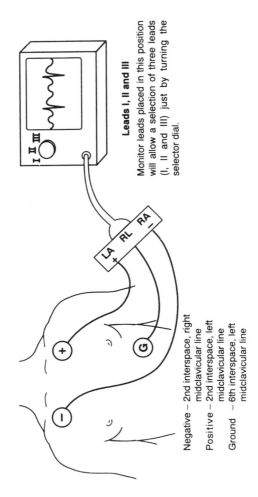

Leads I, II and III

Monitor leads placed in this position will allow a selection of three leads (I, II and III) just by turning the selector dial.

Negative – 2nd interspace, right midclavicular line
Positive – 2nd interspace, left midclavicular line
Ground – 6th interspace, left midclavicular line

Figure 14-3. Electrode and lead placement for bedside monitoring.

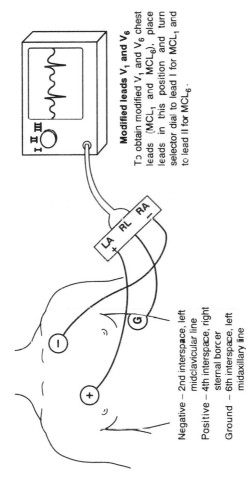

Modified leads V₁ and V₆

To obtain modified V₁ and V₆ chest leads (MCL₁ and MCL₆), place leads in this position and turn selector dial to lead I for MCL₁ and to lead II for MCL₆.

Negative — 2nd interspace, left midclavicular line

Positive — 4th interspace, right sternal border

Ground — 6th interspace, left midaxillary line

Figure 14-3. (continued).

placements, or patient preparation and proper attachment of the electrodes to the skin, refer to Chapters 2 and 5.

Trouble-Shooting Artifacts

One of the primary concerns in cardiac monitoring is distinguishing arrhythmias from artifacts, an artifact being anything other than the heart's electrical activity that causes an ECG tracing. Artifacts cause the monitor's alarm system to trigger. The patient care provider or monitor technician needs to be able to trouble-shoot any alarms, distinguish arrhythmias from artifacts, and intervene appropriately, either responding to the arrhythmia or correcting the cause of the artifact. Some common artifacts are explained below.

BROKEN WIRES AND LOOSE, DIRTY, OR CORRODED ELECTRODES

This artifact, created by equipment, presents a picture of a *wandering baseline* that is accentuated with wavelike patterns. This artifact occurs when the stylus is interrupted during its movement up and down the page. This equipment malfunction can easily be corrected by replacing, repairing, or adjusting the loose/broken wires and the dirty/corroded electrodes.

MUSCLE TREMORS

This artifact creates a picture of jagged peaks of irregular heights and a shifting baseline. The pattern significantly distorts the P wave and QRS complex interpretation. This artifact is caused by involuntary muscular movements (Parkinson's disease, shivering, seizures). This artifact can be corrected if the patient's condition improves.

ALTERNATING ELECTRICAL CURRENT

Alternating electrical current is a type of electrical delivery used by health care institutions for electrical equipment. Sometimes an electrical current will drift away from its primary electrical source and interfere with the electrical conduction of the cardiac monitor. This interference is characterized on the ECG by small, spiked lines on a wide, dark baseline. This artifact can be corrected after accurate problem identification and verification that the ECG machine is correctly grounded.

PATIENT MOVEMENTS

Unintentional movement by the patient creates an artifact caused by involuntary muscular tremors. The characteristic pattern is identified by undefined, widely separated wavelike patterns interspaced with clearly distinguishable P waves and QRS complexes. Sometimes these artifacts cannot be prevented; accurate distinction from an arrhythmia is essential.

Rhythm strips in Figures 14-4, 14-5, and 14-6 illustrate how artifacts from patient movement, equipment problems, and electrical interferences can trigger false rate alarms. Additional reference materials should be used if a more comprehensive analysis is desired.

(text continues on page 255)

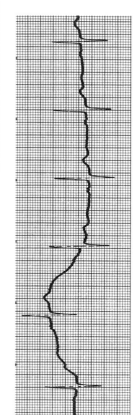

Figure 14-4. Artifacts on ECG pattern caused by patient movement.

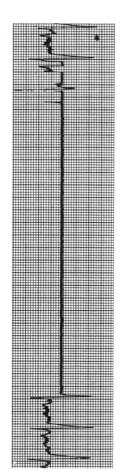

Figure 14-5. Artifacts caused by a loose electrode pad.

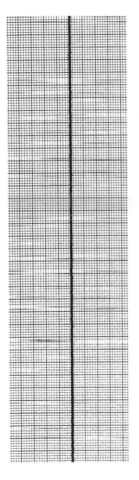

Figure 14-6. Artifacts caused by a disconnected electrode.

Unit Summary

This unit concludes the presentation of pacemaker therapy and continuous cardiac monitoring. ECG patterns commonly seen with pacemakers and caused by artifacts were presented and reviewed. Emphasis was placed on distinguishing expected ECG patterns, trouble-shooting equipment, and distinguishing arrhythmias caused by artifacts from those caused by a cardiac condition.

This unit concludes the book. It is hoped that this "need-to-know" information will help you understand the basics of the ECG and help you identify and distinguish various essential arrhythmias.

Answer Key

Chapter 3

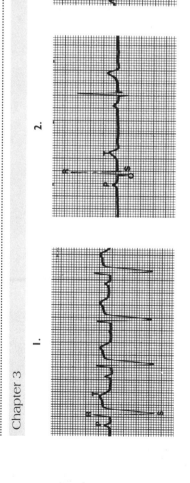

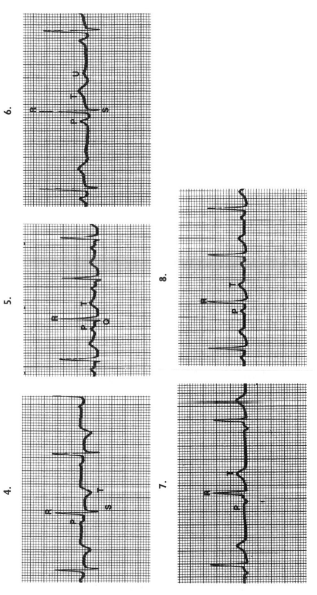

Chapter 4

1. Rhythm: regular
   Rate: 79
   P waves: sinus
   PR interval: 0.14 to 0.16 second
   QRS: 0.06 to 0.08 second
   Interpretation: inverted T wave present
2. Rhythm: regular
   Rate: 45
   P waves: sinus
   PR interval: 0.14 to 0.16 second
   QRS: 0.08 second
   Interpretation: No significant abnormality
3. Rhythm: regular
   Rate: 88
   P waves: sinus
   PR interval: 0.20 second
   QRS: 0.08 second
   Interpretation: depressed ST segment present

4. Rhythm: irregular
   Rate: 50
   P waves: sinus
   PR interval: 0.16 to 0.18 second
   QRS: 0.04 second
   Interpretation: No significant abnormality
5. Rhythm: regular
   Rate: 100
   P waves: sinus
   PR interval: 0.20 second
   QRS: 0.08 second
   Interpretation: extremely elevated ST segment present
6. Rhythm: regular
   Rate: 136
   P waves: sinus
   PR interval: 0.14 to 0.16 second
   QRS: 0.06 to 0.08 second
   Interpretation: No significant abnormality

7. Rhythm: regular
   Rate: 68
   P waves: sinus
   PR interval: 0.16 to 0.18 second
   QRS: 0.12 to 0.14 second
   Interpretation: U wave present
8. Rhythm: irregular
   Rate: 50
   P waves: sinus
   PR interval: 0.12 to 0.14 second
   QRS: 0.08 second
   Interpretation: elevated ST segment and an inverted T wave present

Chapter 6

1. Rhythm: regular
   Rate: 40
   P waves: sinus
   PR interval: 0.14 to 0.16 second
   QRS: 0.08 second
   Interpretation: sinus bradycardia
2. Rhythm: regular
   Rate: 107
   P waves: sinus
   PR interval: 0.14 to 0.16 second
   QRS: 0.08 to 0.10 second
   Interpretation: sinus tachycardia;
   T wave inversion present
3. Rhythm: regular
   Rate: 56
   P waves: sinus
   PR interval: 0.15 to 0.18 second
   QRS: 0.04 to 0.06 second
   Interpretation: sinus bradycardia

4. Rhythm: irregular
   Rate: 50
   P waves: sinus
   PR interval: 0.14 to 0.16 second
   QRS: 0.04 second
   Interpretation: sinus arrhythmia:
   sinus bradycardia
5. Rhythm: regular
   Rate: 60
   P waves: sinus
   PR interval: 0.14 to 0.16 second
   QRS: 0.08 to 0.13 second
   Interpretation: sinus arrhythmia
6. Rhythm: regular
   Rate: 115
   P waves: sinus
   PR interval: 0.12 second
   QRS: 0.08 to 0.10 second
   Interpretation: sinus tachycardia

7. Rhythm: irregular
   Rate: 60
   P waves: sinus
   PR interval: 0.12 to 0.16 second
   QRS: 0.08 to 0.10 second
   Interpretation: sinus arrhythmia
8. Rhythm: regular
   Rate: 115
   P waves: sinus
   PR interval: 0.12 second
   QRS: 0.06 to 0.08 second
   Interpretation: sinus tachycardia
9. Rhythm: basic rhythm regular; ir-
   regular during pause
   Rate: basic rhythm rate is 47
   P waves: sinus in basic rhythm;
   absent during pause
   PR interval: 0.20 in basic rhythm;
   absent during pause

QRS: 0.06 to 0.08 second in basic rhythm; absent during pause

Interpretation: sinus bradycardia with sinus arrest

10. Rhythm: basic rhythm regular; irregular during pause

Rate: basic rhythm rate is 65

P waves: sinus in basic rhythm; absent during pause

PR interval: 0.20 second in basic rhythm; absent during pause

QRS: 0.04 to 0.06 second in basic rhythm; absent during pause

Interpretation: normal sinus rhythm with sinus arrest

Chapter 7

1. Rhythm: irregular

Rate: 70

P waves: fibrillation waves

PR interval: not discernible

QRS: 0.06 to 0.08 second

Interpretation: atrial fibrillation; some flutter waves noted

2. Rhythm: regular

Rate: 188

P waves: hidden in T waves

PR interval: not measurable

QRS: 0.08 second

Interpretation: paroxysmal atrial tachycardia

3. Rhythm: irregular

Rate: 100

P waves: vary in size, shape, and position

PR interval: 0.12 second

QRS: 0.06 to 0.08 second

Interpretation: wandering atrial pacemaker

4. Rhythm: irregular

Rate: atrial = 320; ventricular = 80

P waves: flutter waves present

PR interval: not measurable

QRS: 0.08 second

Interpretation: atrial flutter with variable block

5. Rhythm: irregular

Rate: 70

P waves: vary in size, shape, and position

PR interval: 0.12 to 0.14 second

QRS: 0.06 to 0.08 second

Interpretation: T wave inversion

6. Rhythm: irregular

Rate: ventricular = 110

P waves: fibrillatory waves present

PR interval: not measurable

QRS: 0.06 to 0.08 second
Interpretation: atrial fibrillation; some flutter waves noted

7. Rhythm: regular
Rate: 188
P waves: not identified
PR interval: not discernible
QRS: 0.04 to 0.06 seconds
Interpretation: paroxysmal atrial tachycardia; ST depression present

8. Rhythm: regular
Rate: atrial = 300;
ventricular = 100
P waves: three flutter waves before each QRS
PR interval: not measurable
QRS: 0.08 second
Interpretation: atrial flutter with a 3:1 block

9. Rhythm: regular
Rate: 188
P waves: hidden in T waves
PR interval: not measurable
QRS: 0.04 second
Interpretation: paroxysmal atrial tachycardia; ST segment depression present

10. Rhythm: regular
Rate: atrial = 316;
ventricular = 79
P waves: four flutter waves to each QRS
PR interval: not discernible
QRS: 0.06 second
Interpretation: atrial flutter with a 4:1 block

Chapter 8

1. Rhythm: regular
Rate: 60
P waves: sinus P waves present
PR interval: 0.24 second
QRS: 0.06 to 0.08 second
Interpretation: normal sinus rhythm with first-degree AV block; ST segment elevation and T wave inversion

2. Rhythm: regular
Rate: 115
P waves: inverted
PR interval: 0.08 second
QRS: 0.04 second
Interpretation: junctional tachycardia

3. Rhythm regular
Rate: 45
P waves: sinus P waves present
PR interval: 0.24 to 0.26 second
QRS: 0.06 to 0.08 second
Interpretation: sinus bradycardia with first-degree AV block; ST segment depression present

4. Rhythm: regular
Rate: atrial = 60; ventricular = 38
P waves: sinus P waves not relating to QRS complexes; P waves hidden in QRS complexes and T waves
PR interval: varies greatly
QRS: 0.12 to 0.16 second
Interpretation: third-degree AV block

5. Rhythm: regular
Rate: 84
P waves: sinus P waves present
PR interval: 0.24 to 0.28 second
QRS: 0.08 second
Interpretation: sinus rhythm with first-degree AV block

6. Rhythm: regular, irregular with premature junctional contraction
Rate: 136
P waves: sinus P waves with basic rhythm; P waves hidden with premature junctional contractions

PR interval: 0.12 to 0.14 second
QRS: 0.06 second
Interpretation: sinus tachycardia with premature junctional contractions

7. Rhythm: irregular ventricular rhythm; regular atrial rhythm
Rate: atrial = 65; ventricular = 50
P waves: sinus P waves present; one P wave without QRS
PR interval: progresses from 0.20 to 0.48 second
QRS: 0.04 second
Interpretation: second-degree AV block; type I

8. Rhythm: regular
Rate: 125
P waves: inverted before each QRS
PR interval: 0.08 to 0.10 second
QRS: 0.06 second
Interpretation: junctional tachycardia

9. Rhythm: regular
Rate: atrial = 84; ventricular = 28
P waves: sinus P waves not relating to QRS and hidden in QRS complexes and waves
PR interval: varies greatly
QRS: 0.24 second
Interpretation: third-degree AV block

10. Rhythm: regular
Rate: 65
P waves: inverted before each QRS
PR interval: 0.08 second
QRS: 0.04 to 0.06 second
Interpretation: accelerated junctional rhythm with ST segment elevation

11. Rhythm: regular
Rate: 75
P waves: sinus P waves
PR interval: 0.28 second
QRS: 0.08 second
Interpretation: sinus rhythm with first-degree AV block

12. Rhythm: regular
Rate: 41
P waves: inverted after QRS
PR interval: 0.04 to 0.06 second
QRS: 0.06 to 0.08 second
Interpretation: junctional rhythm

13. Rhythm: regular
Rate: atrial = 96; ventricular = 32
P waves: three sinus P waves to each QRS; one hidden in T wave
PR interval: 0.12 to 0.14 second
QRS: 0.12 second
Interpretation: second-degree AV block, type II

14. Rhythm: regular ventricular and irregular atrial rhythm
Rate: atrial = 90; ventricular = 30
P waves: sinus P waves that have no relationship to QRS; waves hidden in QRS and T waves
PR interval: varies greatly
QRS: 0.12 second
Interpretation: third-degree AV block

15. Rhythm: irregular
Rate: 40
P waves: inverted before each QRS
PR interval: 0.04 to 0.06 second
QRS: 0.08 to 0.10 second
Interpretation: junctional rhythm: ST segment depression

16. Rhythm: regular
Rate: 63
P waves: hidden in QRS
PR interval: not measurable
QRS: 0.08 second
Interpretation: accelerated junctional rhythm

Chapter 9

1. Rhythm: regular
Rate: first rhythm cannot be determined because there is only one QRS complex present; second rhythm has a rate of about 250.
P waves: only one sinus P wave present
PR interval: 0.16 second
QRS: 0.06 to 0.08 second (sinus beats); 0.12 second (wide beat)
Interpretation: sinus beat changing to ventricular tachycardia

2. Rhythm: regular; irregular with premature ventricular contractions (PVCs)
Rate: basic rhythm is 75
P waves: sinus P waves have a

basic rhythm; no P waves found with PVCs; sinus P waves can be seen after the PVCs
PR interval: 0.08 to 0.20 second
QRS: 0.08 seconds (basic rhythm); 0.12 seconds (PVCs)
Interpretation: normal sinus rhythm with two unifocal PVCs

3. Rhythm: nonexistent
Rate: chaotic
P waves: chaotic wave deflections of varying height, size, and shape
PR interval: not measurable
QRS: absent
Interpretation: ventricular fibrillation

4. Rhythm: basic rhythm regular; irregular with PVCs
Rate: 79
P waves: sinus P waves present with basic rhythm
PR interval: 0.16 second

QRS: 0.06 second (basic rhythm); 0.12 to 0.16 second (PVCs)
Interpretation: normal sinus rhythm with paired unifocal PVCs

5. Rhythm: regular
Rate: 250
P waves: none identifiable
PR interval: not measurable
QRS: 0.20 second
Interpretation: ventricular tachycardia

6. Rhythm: chaotic
Rate: not measurable
P waves: absent; any deflections present are irregular and vary in height, size, and shape.
PR interval: not measurable
QRS: absent
Interpretation: ventricular fibrillation

7. Rhythm: regular
Rate: 188
P waves: not identified
PR interval: not discernible
QRS: 0.16 second
Interpretation: ventricular tachycardia; ST segment elevation present

8. Rhythm: cannot be determined; only one complete cardiac cycle
Rate: 56
P waves: sinus P waves with basic rhythm
PR interval: 0.16 second
QRS: 0.04 second (basic rhythm); 0.12 second (escape beats)
Interpretation: sinus bradycardia with two ventricular escape beats

9. Rhythm: irregular
Rate: 100
P waves: fibrillation

PR interval: not measurable

QRS: 0.08 second (basic rhythm); 0.12 seconds (PVCs)

Interpretation: atrial fibrillation with a burst of ventricular tachycardia

10. Rhythm: regular; irregular with PVCs

Rate: 100

P waves: sinus P waves with basic rhythm

PR interval: 0.14 to 0.16 second

QRS: 0.08 second (basic rhythm); 0.12 second (PVCs)

Interpretation: normal sinus rhythm with one PVC

11. Rhythm: regular; irregular with PVC

Rate: 56

P waves: sinus P waves with basic rhythm

PR interval: 0.14 to 0.16 second

QRS: 0.08 second (basic rhythm); 0.12 second (PVC)

Interpretation: sinus bradycardia with one PVC

12. Rhythm: regular

Rate: 100

P waves: sinus P waves present

PR interval: 0.16 second

QRS: 0.16 second

Interpretation: normal sinus rhythm with bundle branch block; ST segment elevation present

Chapter 10

1. Acute inferior wall infarction; sinus rhythm at 82 beats/min with left atrial enlargement, left ventricular hypertrophy

2. Acute lateral wall infarction; sinus rhythm at 95 beats/min

3. Acute inferior and posterior wall infarctions; sinus rhythm at 86 beats/min

4. Acute anterior wall infarction; sinus bradycardia at 47 beats/min

Chapter 11

1. Rhythm: regular
   Rate: 88
   P waves: sinus P waves present
   PR interval: 0.16 to 0.18 second
   QRS: 0.12 to 0.14 second
   Interpretation: normal sinus rhythm with bundle branch block

2. Rhythm: regular
   Rate: 72
   P waves: sinus P waves present
   PR interval: 0.16 second
   QRS: 0.12 second
   Interpretation: normal sinus rhythm with bundle branch block

3. Rhythm: regular
   Rate: 79
   P waves: sinus P waves present
   PR interval: 0.20 second
   QRS: 0.12 second
   Interpretation: normal sinus rhythm with bundle branch block; T wave inversion

4. Rhythm: regular
   Rate: 56
   P waves: sinus P waves present
   PR interval: 0.12 to 0.16 second
   QRS: 0.12 second
   Interpretation: sinus bradycardia with bundle branch block; ST segment depression present

5. Rhythm: regular atrial rhythm; irregular ventricular rhythm
   Rate: atrial = 58; ventricular, about 40
   P waves: sinus P waves present
   PR interval: 0.30 to 0.36 second (escape beat)
   QRS: 0.08 second (basic rhythm); 0.12 second (escape beat)
   Interpretation: second-degree AV block; Mobitz I with one ventricular escape beat

6. Rhythm: regular atrial rhythm; irregular ventricular rhythm
   Rate: atrial = 72; ventricular = 50
   P waves: sinus P waves present
   PR interval: 0.16 to 0.28 second
   QRS: 0.12 second
   Interpretation: second-degree AV block; Mobitz 1; bundle branch block present

7. Rhythm: regular
   Rate: 75
   P waves: sinus P waves present
   PR interval: 0.12 second
   QRS: 0.18 to 0.20 second

Interpretation: normal sinus
rhythm with bundle branch
block; T wave inversion
present

8. Rhythm: regular
Rate: 88
P waves: sinus P waves present
PR interval: 0.20 second

QRS: 0.12 second
Interpretation: normal sinus
rhythm with bundle branch
block

Chapter 13

1. Automatic interval rate: 72
Analysis: The first four beats are
paced beats, followed by one
patient beat and three paced
beats.
Interpretation: normal pacemaker function

2. Automatic interval rate: 84
Analysis: The first three beats are
paced beats, followed by two
patient beats; a pacer beat, and
two paced beats.
Interpretation: undersensing or
non-sensing malfunction

3. Automatic interval rate: 72
Analysis: The first two beats are
paced beats, followed by two

spikes that occur on time but do
not capture, and four paced beats.
Interpretation: loss of capture
malfunction

4. Automatic interval rate: 72
Analysis: No patient beats are
seen; no paced beats are seen.
Interpretation: loss of capture in
the presence of asystole

5. Automatic interval rate: 50
Analysis: The first two beats are
pacemaker induced, followed by
a pseudofusion beat, two patient
beats, and one paced beat.
Interpretation: normal pacemaker function

6. Automatic interval rate: 63
Analysis: The first two beats are
paced beats followed by one patient beat, two paced beats, one
patient beat, and one paced beat.
Interpretation: normal pacemaker function

7. Automatic interval rate: cannot
be determined for sure because
two consecutively paced beats
are not present
Analysis: Strip shows six patient
beats and five loss-of-capture
spikes. No paced beats are seen.
Interpretation: complete loss of
capture

8. Automatic interval rate: 56
   Analysis: The first two beats are
   paced beats, followed by one
   patient beat, one paced beat,
   one patient beat, one paced beat
   that occurs too early, two paced
   beats, and one patient beat.
   Interpretation: undersensing or
   non-sensing malfunction

Figure Credits

Sources:

Catalano JT: Guide to ECG Analysis. Philadelphia, JB Lippincott, 1993

Davis D: How to Quickly and Accurately Master ECG Interpretation (2nd Ed.). Philadelphia, JB Lippincott, 1991

Huff J: ECG Workout: Exercises in Arrhythmia Interpretation (3rd Ed.). Philadelphia, Lippincott-Raven, 1997

Laiken N, Laiken SL, Karliner JS: Interpretation of Electrocardiograms: A Self-Instructional Approach (2nd Ed.). Philadelphia, JB Lippincott, 1988

Smeltzer SC, Bare BG: Brunner and Suddarth's Textbook of Medical-Surgical Nursing (8th Ed.). Philadelphia, Lippincott-Raven, 1996

Thaler MS: The Only EKG Book You'll Ever Need (2nd Ed.). Philadelphia, JB Lippincott, 1995

Chapter 1: 1.1, Huff, p. 3; 1.2, Huff. p. 4: 1.3 a–c, Davis, p. 10: 1.4, Brunner, p. 591.

Chapter 2: 2.1, Davis, p. 57; 2.2, Davis, p. 65; 2.3, Thaler, p. 41; 2.4, Thaler, p. 39; 2.5 Thaler, p. 40; 2.6, Smeltzer, p. 617.

Chapter 3: 3.1, Davis, p. 28; 3.2, Catalano, p. 31; 3.3, Davis, p. 24; 3.4, Davis, p. 59; 3.5, Davis, p. 26; 3.6, Laiken, p. 35; 3.7. Laiken, p. 36; 3.8, Davis, p. 26; 3.9, Huff, p. 17; 3.10, Huff, p. 17; 3.11, Davis, p. 27; 3.12, Davis, p. 25; 3.13, Laiken, p. 28; 3.14, Laiken, p. 29.

Chapter 4: 4.1, Catalano, p. 26; 4.2, Thaler, p. 18; 4.3, Davis, p. 41; 4.4, Catalano, p. 51; 4.5, Catalano, p. 50; 4.6, Davis, p. 39; 4.7, Davis, p. 41; 4.8, Davis, p. 38; 4.9, Davis, p. 39; 4.10, Catalano, p. 59.

Chapter 5: 5.1, Catalano, p. 29.

Chapter 6: 6.1, Davis, p. 41; 6.2, Davis, p. 41; 6.3, Huff, p. 43; 6.4, Catalano, p. 87; 6.5, Catalano, p. 89; 6.6, Catalano, p. 91.

Chapter 7: 7.1, Catalano, p. 105; 7.2, Catalano, p. 106; 7.3, Catalano, p. 108; 7.4, Catalano, p. 110; 7.5, Catalano,

p. 112; 7.6, Catalano, p. 113; 7.7, Catalano, p. 115; 7.8, Catalano, p. 116; 7.9, Catalano, p. 117.

Chapter 8: 8.1, Catalano, p. 133; 8.2, Catalano, p. 136; 8.3, Catalano, p. 137; 8.4, Catalano, p. 138; 8.5, Catalano, p. 140; 8.6, Catalano, p. 143; 8.7, Huff, p. 127; 8.8, Huff, p. 128; 8.9, Huff, p. 129; 8.10, Huff, p. 130.

Chapter 9: 9.1, Catalano, p. 157; 9.2, Huff, p. 168; 9.3, Huff, p. 169; 9.4, Huff, p. 169; 9.5, Huff, p. 170; 9.6, Huff, p. 170; 9.7, Catalano, p. 173; 9.8, Catalano, p. 175; 9.9, Catalano, p. 176; 9.10, Catalano, p. 177; 9.11, Catalano, p. 180; 9.12, Catalano, p. 153.

Chapter 10: 10.1, Davis, p. 193; 10.2, Thaler, p. 215; 10.3, Davis, p. 198; 10.4, Thaler, p. 204; 10.5, Thaler, p. 206; 10.6, Thaler, p. 211; 10.7, Davis, p. 214; 10.8, Davis, p. 218; 10.9, Davis, p. 220; 10.10, Davis, p. 222.

Chapter 11: 11.1, Catalano, p. 231; 11.2, Davis, p. 155; 11.3, Catalano, p. 234; 11.4, Davis, p. 158; 11.5, Thaler, p. 171; 11.6, Catalano, p. 237; 11.7, Catalano, p. 237.

Chapter 12: 12.1, Laiken, p. 143; 12.2, Laiken, p. 141; 12.3, Laiken, p. 144; 12.4, Laiken, p. 146; 12.5, Thaler, p. 249.

Chapter 13: 13.1, Huff, p. 212; 13.2, Huff, p. 212; 13.3, Huff, p. 213; 13.4, Thaler, p. 182; 13.5, Catalano, p. 277; 13.6, Catalano, p. 271; 13.7, Catalano, p. 272; 13.8, Catalano, p. 274; 13.9, Huff, p. 215; 13.10, Huff, p. 215.

Chapter 14: 14.1, Huff, p. 22; 14.2, Huff, p. 23; 14.3, Huff, p. 24; 14.4, Huff, p. 25; 14.5, Huff, p. 26; 14.6, Huff, p. 27.

Credits for Practice Strips: Chapter 3, Huff, pp 19–20; Chapter 4, Huff, pp 35–37; Chapter 6, Huff, pp 47–73; Chapter 7, Huff, pp 89–96; Chapter 8, Huff, pp 131–147; Chapter 9, Huff, pp 179–208; Chapter 10, Davis, pp 224–226; 233; Chapter 11, Huff, pp 179–200; Chapter 13, Huff, pp 217–228.

Answer Key: Huff, pp. 269–270.